THE
COLD
FIX

THE
COLD
FIX

**DRAWING STRENGTH
FROM COLD-WATER
SWIMMING AND
IMMERSION**

SARA BARNES

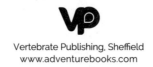

Vertebrate Publishing, Sheffield
www.adventurebooks.com

THE COLD FIX

SARA BARNES

First published in 2022 by Vertebrate Publishing.

 Vertebrate Publishing
Omega Court, 352 Cemetery Road, Sheffield S11 8FT, United Kingdom.
www.adventurebooks.com

Front cover photo: Tom McNally. Other photography as credited.

This book is a work of non-fiction. The author has stated to the publishers that, except in such minor respects not affecting the substantial accuracy of the work, the contents of the book are true.

A CIP catalogue record for this book is available from the British Library.

ISBN: 978-1-83981-158-6 (Paperback)
ISBN: 978-1-83981-159-3 (Ebook)
ISBN: 978-1-83981-160-9 (Audiobook)

10 9 8 7 6 5 4 3 2 1

Cover design, layout and production by Rosie Edwards, Vertebrate Publishing.
www.adventurebooks.com

Vertebrate Publishing is committed to printing on paper from sustainable sources.

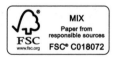

Printed and bound in Great Britain by Clays Ltd., Elcograf S.p.A.

I am broken, but have never felt more whole
Mum, Dad, Emily, Robin and Baloo

CONTENTS

THE TARN

Patchwork black, grey and white mountains loomed in a semicircle around Bowscale Tarn: a mix of black and grey gabbro and granite, white snow and ice. Ravens hiding in deep crevices watched the solitary woman approach the brink of this north-facing tarn and come to a standstill. They waited.

I wanted to catch my breath, gather my thoughts and decide on my entry point. Only I knew why I had stopped. Only I understood how much reaching this point 240 metres up a Lakeland fell on a cold Saturday in December meant to me. Fear of my legs failing me halfway up the snow- and ice-covered bridleway, as they had the previous February because of crippling pain, still haunted me. Lack of confidence to negotiate the icy roads to the start of the bridleway had oozed into me as the road conditions deteriorated. Uneasiness that doing this on my own in the middle of winter was utterly foolhardy had twisted my sense of adventure. But grit and determination to drag myself up on to the next level of physical and emotional recovery had forced a hasty, but considered, packing of my rucksack with essential winter mountain and swimming kit. Then I had swiftly heaved it into the boot of my car before I changed my mind.

Now, on the edge of this eerily quiet, almost holy tarn, I felt humbled. My legs had proved to be strong enough, my fitness levels high enough and the joy I felt in my heart rich enough. All I had to do now was choose the right entry point and check my exit was the same or better. I knew the tarn bed dropped off sharply from the bank, and not surprisingly, this knowledge only fed my fear of deep water. In places, there was what looked like solid ice on the surface so I couldn't see what was below. I reminded myself that this adventure was mostly about completing the walk and less about the swim.

Having said that, my body ached to be immersed in that dark, cold water, to scrunch semi-frozen slush with my bare feet and to feel completely alive on this day of celebration.

A large lump of granite had rolled down the steep mountainside thousands, maybe millions of years ago and its gently sloping shape invited me to rest awhile. It was also in exactly the right place, just beside the tarn's outflow, Tarn Sike. I knew this end was shallow. Suddenly, I felt excited and brave again. Coming here on my own had indeed added a risk factor, but it had also motivated and driven me to climb, literally, out of my comfort zone and rediscover a world that had been out of reach for too long.

Slowly, I stripped off my human layers, folding each piece of clothing carefully in the right order for putting back on when I was frozen post-swim. This deliberate, almost ceremonial, derobing allowed me time to calm my heart rate, breathe more slowly and enjoy the moment. I didn't need anyone else there; I was in a very happy place in my head. To wear neoprene swim socks or not? Life had narrowed to essential decisions only.

Voices broke into my thoughts, and for a moment I felt irritated. I'd planned a solitary, inward-focused experience. I craned my head round to see who was coming up the path: a middle-aged couple with their dog trotting on ahead. The black spaniel ran up to me and sniffed around, but didn't jump up. I had tensed as soon as I saw it approaching me, fearing its claws on my bare legs.

'Morning,' called the woman cheerfully. 'Are you going for a swim?'

To deny my imminent plunge, given that I was just wearing a black swimsuit and a navy bobble hat, would have been churlish to say the least, and although part of me went immediately on the defensive because I didn't want to alarm anyone by swimming alone in winter conditions, the other half leapt into sociable mode, eager to share my passion.

'Yes, just a dip, here, where it's shallow.' I pointed to the black water a short distance from my bare feet, which were now rather cold. I needed to either get in or put some clothes back on.

'Do you mind if I come in with you?' The woman's request took me by surprise and without thinking I responded with an enthusiastic, 'Yes, of course. Are you a swimmer?'

Her husband nodded and raised his eyes skywards. 'She gets in everywhere; I just hold her towel.'

With a smile, I waited by my rock while the woman quickly stripped down to sturdy black sports bra and knickers. Suddenly, my solitary swim had become something else, something actually rather exciting and heart-warming. She was so thrilled to have found me by the tarn, she said, as she picked her way across the frozen grass and loose stones towards me.

I was tempted to take her hand so that we could walk in together, but I hardly knew her! The thought made me laugh and then I counted: one, two, three! In we walked, gasping as the slush grazed our feet and then our calves. So far so good, though – the bottom of the lake here was firm, if a little tricky because of the stones. I closed my eyes for a moment and breathed in deeply, one step closer to relaxing before the cold water bit in as it reached the top of my thighs. Caroline (she'd introduced herself as we were standing on the edge) let out an 'Ooooh!' as her nether regions met semi-frozen tarn. Then it was my turn to gasp, being slightly taller. The shared experience of doing something so ridiculous as walking half naked into water so cold that it could kill you in minutes if you accidentally fell in, did something to normal social filters. In this moment we were connected and nothing else mattered. Her husband and dog stood in silence on the bank, but they may as well have been warming themselves by the fire in the pub, so unaware of them were we.

Our feet were sliding about inelegantly, but we gripped each other to keep balance and then we found the 'boggy bit'! It was each to her own now and in we fell, face-planting the tarn and taking a few panicky strokes before standing up again and shrieking at each other. 'Oh my God! That's cold.'

This place of brooding crags and staring ravens echoed with our chatter and squeals as we each revelled in being there, in having met each other, in sharing this amazing experience. Caroline's husband was taking photographs and I had my GoPro – everything was being recorded digitally and emotionally.

But although I loved what we were doing, a part of me still wanted a few moments in the tarn alone. It was Caroline who said, 'Thank you so much for letting me join you, but don't you want to be here on your own?'

She understood, as swimmers seem to. I smiled and nodded. 'Thank you,' I added.

I felt good, not cold, and I could still feel my fingers and toes. But we had stirred up silt and floating debris with all our bouncing about and I wanted transparent, icy water around my body. Bowscale is one of the clearest tarns I've swum in; the water quality is unequalled, except perhaps by Wastwater. Time to brave the deep! I walked barefoot along the snowy pathway for a hundred metres or so until I reached clear water; so clear that I could see the bottom between the floating pieces of ice.

Excitement bubbled in my belly and once more I was in the moment, resetting my state of mind to accept the water on my skin. This time it felt warmer, which was all relative, of course, considering further out the tarn was completely frozen over. I couldn't wait to sink down and immerse right up to my chin. At that point I closed my eyes and allowed my body to relax as it adjusted once again to the cold. The metallic smell of icy water floated up into my nostrils: I inhaled it until the back of my throat smarted from the cold. Silence surrounded me above and below, or so it seemed, until my ears tuned in to the minute crackles of shifting ice, the faint murmurs of the couple as the woman dressed and sipped the hot drink her husband insisted she have, an occasional breath of air as the wind ebbed and flowed and, to my relief, my own heartbeat.

I don't write a gratitude journal or routinely give thanks when I dip, but that day felt special for so many more reasons than I could have anticipated when I got up that morning. The strength of mind I had needed to even get myself out of the house, let alone walk up the frozen bridleway, felt overwhelming. I was close to tears at what I'd been able to achieve. This was the 'no turning back point' in my journey to rediscovering a physical life in the Lake District.

BEFORE

Out on my bike I felt free and as strong as anyone else I knew. My legs and willpower could take me up Pyrenean cols and mountain passes steadily, never fast, but I always got to the top and felt elated. Descending was even more thrilling because I was never sure whether I'd make it down in one piece – a blip in the road surface and I'd be over the handlebars – descending always played games with my mind.

On an August sunrise, the Giant of Provence hunkered down under a soon-to-be cerulean blue sky, mild and complacent for once. Fortuitous for me as I crept out of the still-sleeping gite in cycling socks, not wanting to disturb my family at this crazy, still-night hour. White cycling shoes in one hand, handlebar bag in the other, I couldn't help but grin to myself at the adventure I had waited so long for. My original plan, for which I had relentlessly trained, was to attempt to climb the mountain by three different routes in the same day and become a member of the prestigious Club des Cinglés du Ventoux (which literally translates as the 'Mont Ventoux Crazy Club'). Each route is approximately twenty-one kilometres with gradients reaching ten per cent as the tarmac climbs through pine forests and open mountain slopes to the summit at 1,910 metres. Success is definitely not guaranteed and many cyclists are forced to submit to the mountain's fierce and unpredictable weather patterns, which are partly down to its geographical position – in the middle of a plain with no other mountain nearby. The so-called 'bald mountain' is a bit of a monster!

But I was ready for a monster of a ride: Malaucène was going to be my first starting point and I already knew how I'd tackle it: plenty of water, a few snacks, a few photo opportunity stops (probably not officially allowed, but in my book I'd still have climbed the mountain and reached the summit) and above all else by zoning out, allowing my mind to travel to a nicer place, leaving my legs, lungs and heart to do the work.

It was how I'd climbed El Tiede, Col d'Aspin and numerous other epic and classic routes around Europe. Distance became irrelevant so long as I allowed myself the above essentials. And it made solo cycling less lonely.

Being zoned out and pedalling steadily in a comfortable low gear were working perfectly and I knew my heart rate was not being pushed anywhere near my limit, but I saw no reason to work harder. Why make it any more painful than it already was? The small white placards every now and again indicating the gradient had remained at seven per cent, but on the way up towards Chalet Renard every fibre of my body knew that the gradient had increased. Sure enough, the next placard grimly reported ten per cent.

Now it was even harder to zone out. My heart rate had increased so that I could hear the blood pulsing through my temples; my fingers gripped the handlebars as if by pushing down I would be propelled forwards faster. My legs ached from the additional effort and even though I dropped a gear or two, nothing seemed to alleviate the pain and urge to unclip and give up. I knew there were four more kilometres at this gradient and if I didn't calm myself down and settle into a relaxed rhythm, I'd blow up.

The hardest battle I'd ever faced on a bike began.

First, I controlled my breathing by consciously slowing it down and deliberately drawing in more air through my nose and blowing it out in long blasts through my mouth. My muscles became more oxygenated and my vision cleared, leaving me free to focus on the tarmac ahead as it rose up and up.

There are no bends on this part of the climb and the road is quite wide. On the left-hand side a few trees protect you from any wind, and on the right is a steep bank of reddy-coloured rock and sand, where road-making machinery has gouged out the mountainside. You can see what lies ahead and it is terrifying.

No respite from the toil of turning the pedals, listening to the scrunch–scrunch of tyres on the hot, dusty tarmac.

Determined to stay seated on the saddle, I chose a gear that I could sustain and forced my mind to journey somewhere else – a shady orchard with a long wooden table laid out ready for lunch. On it were hand-painted ceramic plates, long-stemmed wine glasses, bowls of ripe cherry tomatoes, sweet peppers and grapes. Every time I felt the pain intruding, I added another delicious dish: garlic-scented couscous, pan-fried goat's cheese and delicately dressed green salad leaves.

And that was how I reached the top of the Giant of Provence in my fifty-second year, quite possibly the best cerebrally fed cyclist ever to have conquered the monster.

More importantly, it was the last monster I ever conquered on a bike. Those legs that had powered me up the mountain were breaking down inside, cartilage was being eaten by a disease and pain started to become my daily torturer.

To unravel from this level of fitness and strength and watch myself become increasingly immobile broke me into thousands of pieces, emotionally and physically.

Today, more than five years after surgery, I know that I will never cycle at this level again, I will never have the privilege of calling myself a Mont Ventoux Crazy, but do you know what? Even on that historical August day in 2013, my thought processes had started to change. Halfway up the road from Malaucène, I made the decision to not take on the massive three-way cycle ride I had worked so hard for. Why was I willing to do that? Because it didn't feel right to spend the whole day away from my family, expect them to drive around after me, watch me suffer on the climbs and then to have to put up with me being too tired to join in their fun on what was after all meant to be a holiday. For too many years I had stolen hours from them that could have been 'mum and kids' hours, instead of 'mum obsessively cycling' hours.

What had I been running away from? Because that was the question that had kept me awake the night before my Ventoux Challenge: what was I afraid of if I just stopped, full stop?

STOPPING

I'm alive.

No pain.

Don't feel sick.

Can I move my legs?

Ow!

I opened my eyes and moved my head on the pillow, licking my lips, which were a bit dry, and my throat was sore from being intubated during surgery. I lifted my left hand to look at the intravenous cannula, taped on with a tube coming out of it, feeding me painkillers. My eyes closed again and I sighed, partly out of relief it was over, partly from post-op sleepiness.

Reassuring noises: telephone, voices, various beeps, whirring machines, and one that I didn't recognise, coming from halfway down the bed. That was when I started to drift back into reality. The rhythmic pumping noise was connected to the gentle squeezing and releasing of the cuffs wrapped around my lower legs: they were connected to the Intermittent Pneumatic Compression machine to help prevent DVT. But I couldn't be bothered to lift the sheet to take a peek.

When I signed the yellow consent form to have major surgery on both legs at the same time in February 2017, I had no idea how awful the post-op recovery period would actually be. Nor did I ever imagine that it would be the start of an incredible journey of hope, self-discovery and healing.

At the age of fifty-three I became extremely bow-legged and I could hardly walk. I was diagnosed with severe osteoarthritis in both inner knee joints. Cycling and running had become impossible, places like Mont Ventoux a distant memory. Everyday activities, including cooking, going up and down stairs, doing the washing, gardening and getting in and out of the bath or shower, were excruciating. I lived off painkillers to numb everything and to help me sleep.

My consultant gave me some stark choices. Do nothing, the pain would increase, and my mobility would decrease until I was in a wheelchair anyway. Have one leg operated on at a time and the recovery would be far easier, but possibly take longer.

Or – SNAP, SNAP! – have a bilateral osteotomy and be prepared for short-term pain for long-term gain. There were no guarantees for how successful the operation would be, but he was confident I would get my 'Eureka' moment within six months.

With either procedure, he insisted on my being completely non-weight-bearing for at least eight weeks post-op to allow the broken tibia time to mesh and heal. If I had both legs done at once, I would have to use a wheelchair. To be honest, this didn't really mean anything to me. I had no idea how not being able to bear weight would affect me on a daily basis.

The consultant thought I had the 'right' character to go for the bilateral option. Apparently, because I was athletic and had the mindset to challenge myself physically on a regular basis, he felt I would be able to cope with the difficult recovery. What neither of us knew or even expected was that this 'difficult' recovery would be never-ending.

Back to a chilly, grey Lancastrian afternoon in the hospital, nearly at the end of day one. I thought I'd be allowed out on day four. I'd borrowed two wheelchairs. My plan was to keep one upstairs to move around the large, open-plan kitchen, dining and sitting room, and the lightweight one downstairs to get from my bedroom to the en-suite bathroom.

Gingerly, I lifted the sheet to take a look at my legs. I tried bending them up, but it hurt too much and I winced. How on earth was I going to have a pee? I pressed the buzzer that lay on the bedcovers. After a few minutes, a nurse arrived, smiling and asking what I wanted.

No, hang on a minute, I thought, as she started to help me out of bed. I've just had both legs broken; it's not a good idea to stand up and walk. Hasn't anyone told her that I need to be non-weight-bearing?!

Was it my imagination, or was she overly brusque when I asked her to bring me a bedpan? She didn't seem bothered that I couldn't pee, but suggested I try drinking more water and offered to come back later so we could try again.

What was she going to do? Push down on my bladder for me? I knew from bitter experience that it was not going to work – I could drink my bladder into full capacity, it'd go into shock and I'd need a catheter. They might as well have done it there and then and saved me from all the pain and anguish I knew I'd experience over the next few hours.

But it wasn't until late that night that they relented and the catheter relieved me of 869 millilitres – no wonder the pain in my lower body had become intolerable.

So that was day one. The pain level had gone up to a strong eight out of ten by the time the lights were dimmed and the nurses did their rounds.

As expected, on day four I was allowed home as I'd finally managed to pee all on my own. My daughter had driven down in my mother's car to collect me. Brave, I thought; she was not used to driving an automatic, but we had no other option. I was a little worried about how she was going to manage the wheelchair. I am five foot ten, not light, and she had no experience of this sort of thing. With a little help from the nurses and with me behaving and doing what I was told, I was safely installed in the front passenger seat and Emily squeezed the wheelchair into the back.

It felt so good to be home. It wasn't easy getting the wheelchair plus me up the outside steps into my room, but with Emily, my mother and my son, Robin, all pulling and pushing, we made it. And, by using the bright yellow plastic banana board supplied by the physiotherapist in the hospital, I transferred myself from the wheelchair on to the bed.

But I couldn't stay in bed forever. I was going to have to work out how to get myself around so that I could do basic daily tasks independently. The first and most urgent manoeuvre was from bed to wheelchair to toilet and then from toilet back to wheelchair. And that was when the bond between Emily and me got tested on a new level. This is not something you want anyone else to witness, let alone your daughter. There inevitably comes a time for all parents and their offspring when the roles are reversed, but this was premature and one of the hardest things I've had to do, much harder than exposing your body to the medical profession during pregnancy and childbirth.

Oh God. This recovery was going to be difficult, humiliating and painful.

My every need was going to have to be met by my daughter or my mother. It was just dawning on me how helpless I had become. I did not want anyone to see me naked, sitting on the toilet or struggling to wash myself in the shower sitting on a stool. Thank God every member of my family seemed to be blessed with a down-to-earth sense of humour.

That first evening, post-shower, without any hints or suggestions from me, Emily filled a washing-up bowl with warm water and spa crystals and gave me a foot pamper, which included rubbing spa cream into my feet. I had never had anyone do this for me before. She sat cross-legged on the bathroom floor in front of my wheelchair, and told me to put my feet in the bowl and let her do the washing. Music from her phone wafted in from my bedroom and I allowed myself to be looked after.

My first night was easy; I was still spaced out with a cocktail of drugs, so relatively pain-free. But as this wore off over the next few days I found that it was at night that my mind started to play games with me.

Nothing can prepare you for how awful you feel alone in the night. The weight of your loneliness suffocates you. The yearning for this to be over frustrates you. The fear of the unknown eats away at you from the inside out. I had questions that I was too scared or embarrassed to ask: will anyone fall in love with me again? Will I be able to walk up mountains again? Will I ever cycle up an alpine pass again? And what about sex? I guess I'd better take reverse cowgirl off my bucket list now.

These were dangerous, self-destructive questions that were born out of being scared of the future and what it now held, private questions that I had no one to ask. So I kept them buried deeply inside me and just took more painkillers to bring the relief of sleep. But I knew that when I woke, the questions would surface again.

And then I remembered I had been discharged from hospital with some liquid morphine in case the pain exceeded the reach of all the other painkillers I was swallowing. My mother had jokingly (I think) asked me whether I'd give her the bottle if I didn't use it. 'Just in case,' she half laughed, but I guessed at what she was thinking.

It helped me to sleep.

When I was a little girl, I wrote a short story about being a mouse living on the tracks of the London Underground. I think I'd been influenced by Mary Norton's book *The Borrowers*. My mouse had a daily struggle to keep clean and he was deaf. He scampered about on the tracks searching for titbits, and as soon as he sensed the slightest tremor he jumped down into the dirt and lay as flat as he could, often under a discarded cigarette packet.

I think in the end he misjudged the tremor and got flattened anyway, but that's another story. I have always had a very vivid imagination, so I found it easy to miniaturise myself, grow fur, whiskers, beady black eyes and nimble, pink paws.

The only way I knew how it felt to be an eel, on the other hand, was because I started to dream about them after taking the liquid morphine that night. The dreams were vivid and I was the eel.

In my dreams I could dive down into black water without hesitation, fearless, fast and strong. On the riverbed I wriggled about looking for food, turning over stones and pebbles with my head, flicking my tail to catch up with a fleeing fish or frog. Bored of the depths, I swam up towards the glittering surface of the water, brushing carelessly through lacy weeds. Nothing clung or stuck to my silky smooth body; I was invincible and bold.

As I lost the feeling of weightlessness and speed, I knew I was waking up, coming out of the dream. My brain reconnected to the broken bones in my legs and pain entered my world once more. The heaviness of immobility pressed me into the mattress and I needed to turn over, ease my aching back and hips. The night was over and another day was beginning. But in my dreams I was an eel: vibrant, strong and free.

Given the quirky layout of my house, on several floors with four different flights of stairs, I was confined to my bedroom for eight weeks. Those flights of stairs may as well have been the climb up Mount Everest. And my bedroom was Base Camp. At least I'd got to Base Camp!

Great, I thought, something to keep me busy, and surely it would be relatively easy to achieve the climb up to the kitchen and life as I had once known it? I'd just go up and down on my bum and somehow get into the wheelchair without putting my feet on the floor. And therein lay the problem: if you can't put your feet down, you have to rely on the strength of your arms and upper body. I bought some kettlebells.

In the meantime, I decided to practise on the three steps leading up to the next floor. Emily placed the banana board across from the wheelchair to the second step. Not quite. The banana board only just reached and my arms weren't yet strong enough to bear the weight of my body.

Second attempt.

With careful positioning of the wheelchair, I managed to slide across from the seat on to the banana board and then on to the step. Emily then whisked the banana board plus wheelchair out of the way. It was so tempting to push down with my heels, but I knew I mustn't. I was terrified of snapping my healing broken bones.

We thought for a few minutes about what to do next.

Emily placed an upside-down washing-up bowl with a cushion on top of it under my feet. The idea was for my legs to be relaxed on it, supported rather than under any pressure, which left me free to push down with my hands on to the step behind me. With an enormous heave I succeeded in dragging my bum up and on to the step. As planned, my legs followed me up. Emily moved the bowl back under my feet and I was able to get on to the landing.

I rolled about a bit, relishing just lying flat on the hard, carpeted floor. I called to Robin and my mother, who were upstairs in the kitchen, to come down and see me and share my joy (I learnt later my mother was cross because she thought we were messing about when she needed help getting lunch!). I could chat to my mother and Emily, although Emily was still bustling about and my mother was waiting for Emily to stop bustling before she put the broccoli on. But Emily, being Emily, was still bustling because she didn't think the broccoli was ready yet.

After a few days of hard work, finally I got myself upstairs into the kitchen and living room. Emily dragged the wheelchair up after me so that I didn't have to bum-shuffle across the floor like a tired old slug. We also installed a commode up there, tucked away discreetly by the grandfather clock in the corner. When it struck the hour, I peed.

It was early May 2017; three months post-op, I was now weight-bearing using crutches, but not allowed to drive. Emily had come home for a few days to check on how I was doing. It was a stunning spring day, with real warmth in the sun, but Crummock Water still holds its winter chill well into June. We were going to have a family trip to the lake, said Emily, for a potter and a picnic. I thought I might try and swim because it was something I could do 'without legs'. As a family, we've often swum in the lake and river pools, so neither of my children were surprised, and I was excited when they said they'd join me, but in their wetsuits.

From this end of the lake you can see right down to where Rannerdale Knotts juts out into the water, creating a small, sheltered cove, much loved by divers, swimmers and local teenagers on a summer evening.

Round the corner, Crummock continues and, as you follow the narrow road that teeters just above its dark waters, you can take a peek at the gentle fells of Rannerdale on your left and, on your right, the more rugged, roadless western side, which stretches up to Mellbreak and the lower fells of the High Stile range. After a period of wet weather, Scale Force and other mountain becks thunder down the fells, creating bright, white torrents that cut into the brown-green rocky slopes. I imagine the mountains' hearts have broken and there is no stopping their tears.

My son and daughter's pre-swim warm-ups made me laugh as I lolloped down to the water's edge, using a pair of crutches to help me across the pebbles to where Robin and Emily were strutting like supermodels posing for a new range of wetsuits: 'sun's out, guns out', pouting and flicking their hair.

Dropping my crutches on to the beach, I gesticulated impatiently and urged my children to get ready. 'Come on! Hurry up!' It was pretty nippy standing there in just a swimsuit; I needed to get in the water out of the slight breeze that seemed to have picked up. I was also worried about standing for too long on my half-mended legs without the support of crutches.

Excitement, trepidation, pain and impatience swirled around inside me as I started to walk in; I didn't want to fall or be pushed, but as Robin squealed past me, waving his arms in the way that only teenage boys can, the cold water splashed up on to my bare back and arms and I'm afraid I couldn't hold back some (to use our family term for it) 'non Boxing Day' language.

Satisfied with my reaction, he turned and headed towards his sister.

Emily was cautious too, but mostly because she didn't want to get her hair wet, I thought. She shouted at Robin for splashing her and that's when I noticed she'd got her phone in her hand and was taking selfies – no wonder she was being cautious!

'Come on, Emily, get rid of your phone and let's swim!' I called.

'In a minute,' she responded.

More photos and more hair tossing.

I was up to my thighs now, embracing the chilli-pepper prickles popping wildly on my skin. Looking down through the clear water at my poor, scarred legs, I felt detached from them; they were no longer the focus of my world.

I breathed in deeply. Mossy, clean, soothing aromas filled my lungs: the water, the stones, the silty lakebed, the budding leaves dipping into the water.

My senses came alive.

Standing alone, in a world of my own, I trailed my hands delicately across the surface of the water, drawing a wide circle as my waist twisted from side to side. I could feel my body again, the way it wanted to move, pain-free, flexible and strong, just like the eel I had dreamt of.

A shudder passed down my back and I was brought back into the now.

I wanted someone else near me. As I stepped forward I could see that the water was getting deeper. And then dropped into dark. I don't like seeing that. I have an innate fear of deep water. It's about what else is in the water with you.

Robin came splashing back towards me with a wicked grin on his face and I knew that unless I immersed myself in the next second or two I was going to get pushed in. Just before he could reach me, I bent my knees and down I went.

I tried to relax my breathing as the cold bit into my core. Swearing and gasping threatened to take over as my whole body fought to defend itself. My son sploshed in next to me and I pushed him away, reminding him not to kick at my legs. Then there was Emily too, her hair piled on top of her head, grinning as she swam a graceful heads-up breaststroke towards us.

As we headed out into open water, I tried to quash the fear rising from my stomach and the dark thoughts that crawled out from the corners of my mind.

My imagination was kicking in and I was quite glad when Robin distracted me with a splash and a wriggle as he tried to touch the bottom. But he couldn't, so panicked and half swam, half splashed his way back to where he could stand – and then ran out. I turned round too, a little panicky myself, but Emily was calm and her presence reassured me.

I relaxed and could breathe normally. I floated on my back and looked up at the sky. Immediately, I felt composed and could refocus on my surroundings.

It was one of those days where the clouds floated freely, forming shapes high above me. The mountains and fells were a bright green in their spring clothes. Mellbreak, Grasmoor and Whiteside were all cloud-free and I was sure I could touch them.

I forgot where I was.

My legs floated out in front of me, pain-free. I didn't want to get out and have to put weight on them again, not just yet. In that moment, the water whispered something insane to me: it would help me on my journey back to full mobility. I didn't need to ask how. I just knew it to be true.

It took until May 2020, three years from that first swim in Crummock, for me to get some pain-free days, to walk again with a 'normal' gait, to finally begin to believe that I had a physical future. Three years of daily physiotherapy, on my own or with a sports therapist; three years of all-season swimming in the lake; and three years of training myself to withstand the bite of the cold as I walked into the water.

Time to fall in love: with the water that was healing me and with the woman I was rediscovering inside my broken, hurting body.

I went through a difficult stage of having nightmares before each swim. I had to fight an internal battle: did the beach shelve gently down into the lake, or was there a steep drop-off and I'd be in God knows what depth of water? What else was swimming in there with me? Would it see my white legs dangling down? Not a chance! I *never* let my legs dangle – they're either kicking or curled up close to my body.

Those nightmares were worse if I was doing a winter night swim. I remember one particularly difficult occasion when I was meeting a friend for a mid-November dip. As I drove down the road that snakes close to the enormity of Crummock Water, the black hulk of Rannerdale Knotts threw a shadow over the water. Once parked up in the divers' car park, I got out of the car and waited for my friend. Looking up, I saw that more stars had broken free and it felt more comforting to look at them than the water I was about to submit to. Once my friend arrived, there was no turning back.

The air temperature was about 5 °C and the water in this, the deepest part of the lake, might just about have struggled to reach 5°.

There were a few large stones underwater to negotiate and the drop-off was, to put it politely, extreme. I had to commit to the water, stagger briefly and then swim. I tried not to swallow too much of the lake as my breathing sharpened, my legs found nothing below them, my arms didn't seem to have any pull to them and the fears started to flap like vampire bats in my imagination.

I could see my friend's head and shoulders moving out beyond where the ledges jutted out from the Knott. Already I knew that the expanse of cold, deep water between us was just too great for me to cross.

Who knew what was down there, thirty metres below me? Divers had once found a man's body there, his coat pockets weighted down with rocks, a note left in his parked car, 'Body in't lek'.

I couldn't do it.

I stopped, but didn't dare let my legs hang down.

The only things keeping me up were my tow float and the straining muscles in my neck and running across to my shoulders. Otherwise, I was literally petrified. My legs were tightly curled up. My arms waggled about uselessly across the top few inches of water.

'You alright?'

My companion's voice sounded distant, but near enough to shake me from my dangerous state of immobility. I could see her head torch glinting, so I knew she was looking right at me and I could hear the concern in her voice.

'Yes, yes, I'm fine.'

I think now, in hindsight, finding my voice gave me something tangible to hang on to in that black nothingness. I told myself that most swimmers find night swims difficult, especially when it is freezing in the water. But that night it was so cold that it almost didn't feel like water, more like hot pepper clouds – weightless and prickly as my fingers passed through it and I almost (but only for a fragment of a nanosecond!) forgot where I was, not even consciously trying to steady my panting breath. I was awestruck by the feeling, the smell of the water, the deep darkness in which I was floating.

Above, the sky was bursting with white dots, slightly fuzzy where millions of stars nudged close together, and the deep dark indigo spaces in between seemed to shrink the more I stared. I had never seen so many stars, nor been so aware of my senses. Was this what it was like in a flotation tank? Total immersion? I wanted to lie there forever. I really had no concept of being in water. I could have just sunk down, down, down, right to the murky bottom.

I shuddered and swam back to the shore, until I was in water as shallow as I could possibly be in without beaching myself.

My children often tease me about what I would be if I were an animal – a manatee or dugong, apparently. Often mistaken by sailors for mermaids, I always reply in my defence.

Secretly, I've read up on these mysterious creatures. They're marine mammals of the family called *Sirenia*, hence the first sailors were persuaded that manatees were sirens or mermaids. These enormous, and highly intelligent, vegetarians can be found in warm, coastal waters from East Africa to Australia – but rarely in the cold, deep and dark waters of the Lake District.

But tonight, under a now-bold full moon, a star-filled sky and in the shallows of the scariest part of Crummock Water, an adult female, beautiful in her own way, rootled about amongst the algaed rocks and pebbles, searching for something and nothing. She floated on her back, staring up at the crinkly crags of Rannerdale Knotts, and drank in the shine of the moon, while her friend swam alone out in the depths.

Not a sound disturbed the swimmer and the mermaid, each cocooned in thought and no thought, emotions and no emotions, the ebb and flow of their internal tides calming and transforming.

As the months passed and clearly the operation had not been as successful as the consultant would have liked, it became increasingly important to my sense of well-being to get into the cold water. There, I felt no pain. Once immersed, I no longer had to lug around what felt like my 'useless' body.

Out of the water, I had issues with my body, not just in terms of mobility, but the reflection in the mirror told me I was now shaped like a man – an upside-down triangle. Wide shoulders, no waist and narrow hips.

The shape of me was not the shape I was before the operation. The top of my thighs had never touched before, but now when I walked I could feel thigh on thigh – right at the top. I always used to have a gap there – someone once told me it was sexy.

It was not that my legs had got fatter, but that the operation had realigned my legs so they were now straight down from top to toe. Prior to surgery, all my weight had been going down the inside knee joint and bone had been rubbing on bone with no cartilage left to cushion them – pain beyond belief.

Muscle mass and definition had gone from my buttocks, but unevenly. My right buttock had virtually disappeared. My running partner and I had once agreed to shoot each other if either of us got a mono bum. Where was she now when I needed her?

I thought of all the hours I'd been spending at home and, latterly, in the gym, exercising to try and rebuild the soft tissue that was now adjusting to my new alignment: quads, hamstrings, Achilles, ligaments, skin and every fibre of both legs below the knee.

Wild swimming was the treat at the end or beginning of a tough day of gym, exercises and generally moving around, still in pain. If I dosed myself up on painkillers first thing in the morning, I was usually pain-free long enough to tackle more remote locations, but the price I paid was having to spend the rest of the day lying on the sofa, unable to move. But on these occasions my natural adventurous spirit was released, so it seemed worth it.

Anyone's journey into the world of cold-water swimming is slow and sometimes painful on many levels, not just the obvious physical one. Over subsequent winters I learnt how my body reacted to cold water at different times of day, in different locations and under different circumstances and in different emotional states.

Black Moss Pot is located around one and a half miles up a fairly level but rough track from Stonethwaite, a tiny cluster of white-painted cottages with small, lightless windows and protective porches. Stonethwaite Farm was once owned by Fountains Abbey, and prior to that by various religious orders, until it was sold to the National Trust.

A couple of friends and their dog, Poppy, and I followed Stonethwaite Beck and passed through twisted old oaks and larches that clustered around the rocky banks, forming a golden tunnel of autumnal beauty, set against a backdrop of dark-green, mossy stone walls, pink and grey pebbles and stones, white, rushing water in mini waterfalls, and distant craggy outcrops which drew us on up the valley.

The sound of roaring water led us down to the river on our left, enticing that part of us that wanted adventure and icy water on our limbs. We reached Galleny Force, a chasm filled with gin-clear water that was a translucent green-blue as it caught the last few remaining green leaves on the trees overhead, the blue of the sky and every shaft of light that reached into its depths. But we didn't stop there, although it was tempting. A swim in these waters would have been lovely, but something more exciting and daring awaited us if we walked another mile and hung on to our anticipation.

Without a signpost to guide us, we just kept to the path as it turned to the right and we were now following Langstrath Beck across a more open, treeless landscape, which felt rough, rugged and wild. There was no sound, except the crunch of boots on moving stones and a slight huff and puff of effort through walking and carrying swim bags and swim cloaks.

It was as if we had lost our way and we wondered whether it might have been prudent to have swum in Galleny Force after all and then sauntered back to the welcome tastes and smells of The Langstrath Country Inn back down in Stonethwaite. Underfoot it was wet and spongy, masses of tiny streams and water paths ran free under the spiky grass and sphagnum moss, and our efforts were channelled into not sinking and getting wet boots and socks.

I looked up and in the near distance there was a house on the crag on the left. Who lived there? Trolls, goblins or the wild men and women of the Jaws of Borrowdale? Then, as we trod closer, the walls and windows of the house crumbled into hard Lakeland rock and colourful lichen and heather. Was it Heron Crag? Sergeant's Crag or Lamper Knott? And just a short way further on we saw a fence straddling dark grey rocks and we knew we were nearly there.

Our natural inclination was to pass through the gate into a flock of sturdy Herdwick sheep, munching hay that the farmer had brought up earlier in the day. Forgetting the nagging pain that had started in my legs, I felt re-energised and my stride lengthened. That first sight of Black Moss Pot shocked me and gave me vertigo. This was a serious chasm: water-filled, steep-sided with black, slimy, inescapable sheets of rock. The sound of thunder overtook any conversation; water is so loud when forced in quantity through a narrow channel of unforgiving rock. So this was where the youth of Keswick playfully jumped in on hot summer days?

We walked back across to the gate and made our way to the other end of the Pot, about fifty metres downstream. Here, the bank provided easier access to the water and the thundering roar was softened by distance, overall a far less intimidating place. The wind had picked up, as it often did when we were about to take off our clothes at the water's edge. It felt bizarre to be stripping down to swimming costume and swim shoes when the 'clag' was shrouding the crags at the head of the valley and we knew we only had a tiny window of opportunity before the weather turned.

I didn't think I'd ever really wanted to swim there; the name itself had always put me off: Black Moss Pot – it looked like it sounded – but here I was on a late October morning not quite 'feeling it'. I had got too warm walking up here, and as I stripped off my layers they felt wet with sweat and my skin was wet too. The wind seemed to know this and found a way of cooling me down, which was not welcome when I was about to swim in cold, river-pool water.

Goggles were essential, as the beauty of this place lay under the water. Finally, we were ready and climbed down using smooth boulders and stepped into Langstrath Beck. Clear, cold and, today, not too fast-flowing. Not too bad! Our swim shoes provided a false sense of security. The temperature was significantly lower than Crummock Water, and my body reacted immediately as I immersed myself in the flow and put my head under the water. Faster breathing, a natural instinct to gulp air, which was actually now water, and I had to stand up again, coughing, calming myself, and then under I went again. I wished I'd put my swim cap on – a protective layer of silicone would definitely have been beneficial that day.

My friend had her GoPro and we tried to pose together on a rock, but slid off and into the water again. The GoPro's real advantage was to allow us to take underwater photos, and I swam along and then sank right down, blowing out bubbles that rose above my head to the surface of the beck. Later, looking at this photograph, it was astonishing to see how the veins on my arms bulged, the flesh on my face was taut and I had taken on the scaly look of a strange fish.

We swam upstream towards the ever-narrowing rocks on either side. Down under the water it was a lot less dark, less scary, but even more dramatic. The colours of the pebbles in the centre of the beck were rose, terracotta, grey and cream; on either side, dark, slippery, shadowy rocks and cliffs squeezed in with menace.

The brightly coloured riverbed dropped down a couple of feet at a time and we were in deeper and deeper water. I forgot to breathe; I didn't realise that the painful, tightening band around my head was not the strap of my goggles but the effects of the cold water – brain freeze – something I'd not experienced before.

But this swim of discovery was addictive and seemingly endless. Once more, we clung together on a ledge to one side and tried to take a few selfies to prove we'd been there. Then we went on, wanting to see what was round the corner. Sense warned us that the water was too cold to continue right up to the end and we didn't know for sure how much further it was. And there was no easy escape. Reluctantly, we allowed our now aching-from-cold bodies to drift back down to lighter, shallower waters. Our feet went down and we stood up, feeling a bit light-headed and giddy. Time to get out.

It was hard work to keep upright on those slippery rocks and as each second passed, my cold blood was pulsing back through my system and my core was cooling down fast. I knew I had to get dried and dressed as quickly as possible. First, I had a few gulps of the hot tea I'd brought with me in a thermos flask, but it was not piping hot. It wouldn't do the job. I fumbled to pull on my microfibre changing robe and released my clammy shoulders from my wet swimming costume. What did I need to do first? I tried to find my underclothes in my swim bag; my knickers had disappeared, but I felt the straps of my bra and pulled it out. As I passed it through the exaggerated armholes of my changing robe, I couldn't remember how to put a bra on. This had never happened to me before.

I felt slightly sick and had to tell myself to stop doing what I was doing. 'Drop the bra, pat yourself dry, try another drink, find your knickers, sit down on that nice round rock, pull your knickers on, but they are stuck to your still-wet legs and bum.' My head felt funny and I could almost hear things moving around inside it, sluggishly and strangely.

'Keep talking. Keep moving. Keep patting and keep rubbing.' I had to force my system to do what it needed to do, to ignore the 'healthy' glow of my swim tan and be aware of what was going on inside my body. I was a little scared, I had to admit. If this was how the after-drop started, then I was concerned. We were a long way from help and I didn't want this pleasant adventure to turn into an epic. I'd drunk all my tepid tea, eaten a pain au chocolat and a banana, but still I wasn't recovering as quickly as I usually did. I saw my friend had poured two mugs of steaming coffee, one for her and one for her husband. I heard myself ask if I could have some.

It was strong and very hot – I could feel it flowing down inside my gullet and hitting the ice-cold pit of my stomach. That started to do the trick. It triggered my system again – and slowly the combination of really hot drink, some food, warm, dry clothing and walking up and down on the spongy sphagnum moss saved me going into full-blown after-drop. Feeling steady enough to walk back up to the fence and lean as far as I dared into the chasm of the Pot, I took some photos with my phone and began to actually look around me at where we were: the tapestry of colours, the hideously broken rocks of the crags where ravens breed and the immortal contours and skyline.

We had both swum somewhere new for each of us; we had immersed ourselves in a moment of landscape and imprinted a memory on our souls.

But even though I learnt a valuable lesson that day, you are always treading a fine line every time you swim in cold water. A few months later, I got very close to mild hypothermia post-swim once more.

It often felt colder to swim in the morning, I had decided, because usually when I set off from home I am still in a cosy state of being snuggled under the duvet and that cosiness doesn't fade gently when I walk into the water. That day, I was hauled out of it wincing and swearing as the cold water bit into my thighs, my 'ooh' zone, my belly. All I could think of was the intense pain as my brain screamed at me to get out, save myself, stop whatever I was doing and run away from danger.

And before I knew it, everything changed. My extremities had lost all feeling and were slowing down. My nostrils flared as I caught the faint scent of clean, cold water; my fingers trailed a little more languidly as I drifted my hands back through the top six inches of glassiness. Giving in to temptation, I rolled on to my back and used my tow float for additional buoyancy.

The sky opened up above me, the wintery tops of the mountains clung on to snow and stared back down at me; a pair of horny drakes competing for a single female winged past me, and I didn't really care what was underneath me … a dangerous, dreamy state … and then, slowly, as a delicious tomatoey pizza hit my stomach, I was able to refocus and realised I was not still in the water, but was back at home, nearly five hours post-swim, in the shadowy lands of mild hypothermia and becoming human again.

To complete the warming-up process I knew it was now long enough after being so cold to be safe to heat through more quickly, so I ran a hot bubble bath, lit some candles and told my son I was going for a soak, to which he grunted and disappeared into his room for some FIFA time. I added some Bio-Oil to the water too.

These indulgent bath soaks had become a bit of a habit for me a couple of hours after a swim or at the end of the day. I listened to music on my phone and allowed it to take me to another place. I lifted a leg out of the bubbles and remembered how I used to be able to point my toes and have such a long, straight leg, no scars, no slightly bent fat knee that still hurt if I tried to force my leg flat. I ran my finger across the longest horizontal scar that was now white; it felt knobbly and stung a bit. How long did it take for flesh to completely heal?

Bringing my knee closer to my head, I rubbed quite hard down my shin, feeling the other lumps and bumps that were still there under the skin – soft tissue, scar tissue, all stuff that needed time to recover. With both hands I massaged my calf, my shin, my ankles and my foot, and then tried to wobble my kneecap. It didn't move at all. So I sat up, bubbles clinging to my shoulders and breasts. With my legs as flat as they would go on the bottom of the bath I pushed down firmly with both hands and released, pushed and released. Each time my leg seemed to lie flatter and the pain lessened. And then I did the same to the other leg. I sighed and flopped my head down on to my chest, peering down at the hated folds in my stomach. God, this was hard work.

One day, in the winter before the world went into pandemic lockdown, I went to a special place because the snows had melted, the hours in the day were drawing out and I felt the need to reconnect and immerse myself in the beauty of this land.

Spirit Pool is a ten-foot-deep gash in the rocks, filled with astonishingly clear, ice-cold water that gushes down from Styhead Tarn in the North-West Lakes. Styhead Gill tumbles past clusters of conifers, rain-gouged grooves in the earth, flood-tumbled boulders and the curiously chewing Herdwick sheep who live there.

You rarely see anyone swimming in this pool and at certain times of day it is a place of watery solitude. At other times you can look up towards the footpath at the garishly clad walkers bent double under the weight of their rucksacks, excited to be on their way up to Scafell Pike, or subdued on their weary way back down, keen to get back to their cars, kick off their boots and find the nearest pub. Very few of them look down towards the gill.

The sheep drink the water at the edge of the river and rarely venture near the rocky outcrops that overhang the pool. For those families who know about it, Spirit Pool is an idyllic place to linger on a hot summer's day, picnic devoured and mind calmed by the sound of bubbling water. For wild swimmers, a few days after a storm, it is a gushing, tumbling, free-falling pool of heaven that takes your breath away and leaves you reinvigorated and bold.

It was a balancing act of courage and nimble-footedness to navigate the slippery stones and boulders in the river shallows, to calm myself before sliding down deep into the embrace of the pool and trying not to cry out at the sting of the cold. Then I succumbed to its magic, the intensity of sensations: the smell of cold water, the sharp nudge against rocks, the mountain orchestra drowning out my thoughts, the taste of moss-peppered bubbles, glimpses of mackerel skies blue above green.

Under the drag of the swirling waters, large boulders hunkered down and it was tempting to swim down head first towards them and reach out to stroke their solid mass. The bite of the cold water on my skin was intensely painful, the flesh of my cheeks contracted and my lips peeled back in a grin. The colours under the water were incredible, a mix of pinks, greys and creams, with a swathe of dark browns and greens where time and weather-dependent water levels have coated the rocks with moss and algae.

At first it was impossible to control where my body was going, because of the sheer force of eddies, swirls and currents all around me. But once I had recovered from the initial exhilaration, I noticed that the left-hand side was relatively slack water, so I swam close to the overhanging jumping-rock, edging towards the dark lip of rock at the head of the pool. This took effort and power; the cold water had intensified my sensations, but gradually sucked away my energy.

Standing up on the lip of the pool, knee-deep in bubbles, I breathed in slowly and then went again – swooshed down in the currents, shrieking and squealing with joy.

It felt so good just to rock myself in its savage cradle, laugh right into the eye of the storm, swim in the slipstream and float back down to the edge of infinity. With a mind full of obstacles, a day brimming with chores, this place washed me free and brought me back to myself, as a child dances back to its mother without a care in the world.

Driving home with a raw sense of hope surging through my veins, I set myself new goals for the year ahead, unaware at that point that for much of it I would be living an increasingly isolated life. First, we all found our freedoms curtailed during a series of national lockdowns during the Covid pandemic and then, just as the world was opening up again, the one person in my life who loved me unconditionally – my mother – became seriously ill and died. I was pitched into the reality of grief.

It was ironic really that, against the backdrop of everything going desperately wrong, I got my legs back. Having been virtually written off by the consultant as a 'less than successful story', I flipped everything on its head and learnt to run in order to be able to walk properly. The Couch to 5k app was a national lockdown phenomenon and for nine weeks I diligently obeyed Michael Johnson's velvety tones as part of my permitted daily exercise. Every Tuesday, Thursday and Sunday for nine weeks, there I was, moving around the local lanes, drawing on every ounce of self-belief and aching every night. But I knew it was working. The communication between my brain and my legs was fizzing back into life, nerves excitedly reconnecting and muscle memory growing plump and proud. My right buttock even began to feel sexy again and I dared to believe one day it would be caressed and gripped in passion by that man who was just waiting somewhere in the water for me.

I completed the challenge a few weeks after my mum's funeral. Ironically, the two things – running and swimming – which had kept me going emotionally and physically during her brief five-week fight with cancer were also the two things she had always worried the most about me doing: the running because she thought it had been my high levels of activity that had exacerbated the osteoarthritis in my knees, and the swimming because she was terrified I would drown. Nothing I could say had ever convinced her that cycling and trail running had not had a negative impact, and I had once promised her that I would always use a tow float when swimming in Crummock Water.

After her death, I remember going into the water without my tow float a couple of times. On both occasions, I had walked back out, unable to swim. It was as if my mum was there in the water with me, watching me, frowning because I was unprotected and unsafe. Such is the power of love.

One afternoon, during the spring following Mum's death, I lay at full stretch in the living room ready to do my daily exercises, which I'd decided to continue in spite of now being far more mobile and relaxed about the state of my legs. The wool rug was beginning to make my back itch, but I was enjoying looking up at the beams and the cobwebs that wafted in the unseasonably warm breeze coming in from the open patio doors. The only sounds were birdsong, the gentle murmur of my neighbours chatting on their patio, the scrunch of gravel as the postman reversed up the track to save turning round.

This room is vast, open from floor to ceiling as barn conversions often are, with Velux windows above my head in the sitting room area. The kitchen is down the other end, with a tall window that looks out over the Western Fells, Skiddaw often in full view. My patio doors lead straight out into the back garden and I can sunbathe here in complete naked privacy, until the neighbour to my right thinks it is a good moment to rootle about with the discarded plastic plant pots and troughs behind his shed. I hang a double sheet over two garden chairs to block his view through the slatted fence.

In the warm sunshine I drifted off to another time when I had thought I was in a room like this. Only that time it hadn't been a real room, but a space created by my imagination and the power of hypnotism.

When I had confided in a friend a handful of years ago that I thought I needed some help dealing with an emotionally abusive relationship, she had recommended a Dutch hypnotherapist in Cockermouth.

In the first session the therapist had suggested that while I was under hypnosis she would guide me back through my life and ask me to think about the different facets of myself, to really probe deep into my psyche: needs, wants, fears, hopes and dreams. She guided this session by asking me questions about my life, and as different experiences and events showed up she tweezered out the emotions and thoughts surrounding them. I had a pen and paper on the table because I had spoken about how I often thought of things in a very visual way, so maybe I could draw what I felt. It turned out that I drew five different characters that represented everything about me. It didn't seem bizarre at the time and I found it easy to see them: a nine-year-old girl with a shy frown, all lanky legs and arms; a large, sleek cat with pantheresque grace and allure; a shadowy, crouching old lady who scuttled from corner to corner; a tall, brazen, long-haired androgynous warrior figure; and, finally, a plumper, older woman with her hair in a messy bun, wiping her floury hands on her jeans and laughing with her eyes.

Afterwards I looked at the pictures and realised that every part of me was there on the paper, but I didn't know what to do with them. 'They are your family,' said the hypnotherapist.

In the next session she told me to go to my happy place, where I felt light-hearted and strong, and once there to sit and wait. So I sat on a sloping beach, the pebbles loosening then settling around my bum cheeks, my legs drawn up to my chest, my arms wrapped round my knees. I watched the light on the sea, glistening and sparkling, ever-changing as the gentle waves lapped the wet strip where the shingle gave way to washed sand. It was beautiful and I was there, right there.

Out of the corner of my eye I glimpsed a dark shape right down on the waterline. I squinted into the sun, trying to make out what it was. Behind it were four other figures. I could recognise them from the way they moved. A skinny young girl was dancing in and out of the waves next to a large, big-pawed cat, trying to grab its tail; a hunched-over figure awkwardly criss-crossed the strands of seaweed; behind her was a woman wearing a long dress which she held up out of the water, jumping over the waves every now and again in bare feet; and finally, a little distance behind them, an incredibly tall, long-haired warrior was striding easily across the sand.

The hypnotist had said, 'Now go down and greet them; they want to meet you.' As I walked slowly across the shifting pebbles, being careful not to fall, I watched the little group turn to stare at me. As I approached, they moved apart slightly and allowed me into the centre of their circle. She was right. I knew these characters already. They were indeed my family, the facets of me that I could call on to help me in different situations.

With this knowledge now imprinted on my brain, the hypnotist went further into my psyche, digging right back to when I was in my mum's womb. The sessions were exhausting, but began to help me make sense of a lot of questions I'd always had, but no one had known how to answer, or didn't want to answer.

Towards the end of this journey, having been stuck in a few dark places, which the hypnotist talked me out of, I walked down a path that seemed wider and the light much brighter. I sensed there were forks off this path that could lead into frightening places, but she asked me if I wanted to go there, or to keep walking down the main path. She asked me how I imagined my ideal life to look, how I would like to be spending my time, who I wanted around me.

'Like this,' I answered, 'lots of light, big white walls where I can hang my paintings, a gentle, warm breeze coming in from the garden, the sound of running water, the people I love relaxing quietly in the sun, eating and drinking, not alone'.

Then she woke me up. 'You already have what you need to find that place, to be safe and happy.'

Did I? Maybe this house, tucked away down a track in a little village in west Cumbria, was that place? It had kept my family and me safe for a few years now, but I didn't love it, I hadn't bonded with it. I still felt I was on a journey and I knew this house didn't feel like the family hub I had hoped it would be. In hindsight, I realise she wasn't referring to the physical house, but to the tools I have within myself and had not yet been able to access.

Back to me lying on the scratchy rug. I made myself dig deep into what was holding me back from reaching that amazing place, why whatever I did just didn't seem to be working. It felt as if there was just too much 'stuff' that was in limbo and I was trying desperately to hold it all in a neat pile in my arms, but bits kept jumping back out again. I'd set so many things in motion, been really positive about all aspects of my life, but I just couldn't move forwards. It felt like something was pinning me down, trapping me, holding me exactly where it wanted me until the time was right.

You know when you're trying to thread a needle and you have to keep licking the fluffy bits on the end, but then the wet bit bends up against the eye, so you lick the thread again? But just as you think it's going through, you drop the needle and bang your head on the cupboard door you left open. Hot tears obscure your vision and you can't find the thread because it's stuck to the bottom of your sock and you need a wee and it's all too difficult.

Life gets like that sometimes.

Blood moons, blue moons, full moons, lunar eclipses. The moon touches something modern society is unable to reach, something twenty per cent of our bodies is unable to connect with. The remaining eighty per cent longs to flow with the push and pull of the tides. This longing will never leave us, but we have subdued it, tried to replace it by living our lives in complicated daily routines.

We peer at our time-starved, stretched-to-the-limit faces in the mirror every morning when we do our teeth, but avoid looking at the longing staring back at us.

We stack our precarious layers of acquisitions, friends, contacts, catalogues, techy stuff and scented candles, until we feel safely surrounded by teetering towers. On top of each precious tower, we then lovingly place a carefully worded To Do list. There we are. Invincible.

It takes but a whisper of breeze, someone walking by, a bird's wings, a door slamming, and those lightweight lists flutter and fall. We tiptoe around the circle of towers, hardly daring to breathe or jump for joy.

And then we see the conundrum we have created. Like an ageing game of Jenga, it's become impossible to slide any single layer out of the tower. We tap it, we wiggle it, we pout and furrow our brows and try again. But too many sticky fingers have touched it, bacteria have grown in the sugary deposits and a noxious layer of glue refuses to let it go.

Those teetering towers trap us within the circle and the longing in eighty per cent of our bodies cries and grieves.

It yells at us to go and swim in ice-cold water, lit up only by the stars and the moon.

Since the beginning of the first national lockdown in the UK in March 2020, I have dipped or swum every day, perhaps without even realising that I have been drawn as if by magic to colder and colder water. It is like nothing else I have ever tried recreationally or athletically. It's not just the natural high I feel afterwards, or the fact that it has given me back my physical mobility and allowed me to rebuild my self-confidence and become an integral, valued member of the global cold-water swimming community. I can't quite put my finger on why it has become so addictive. Why do I feel compelled, whatever the weather, to dip at least once a day, usually in the coldest water I can find? And what compels other dippers, plungers, swimmers and dunkers to do likewise? How does it make other people feel? How has it changed their lives? It began to dawn on me that there could be a thousand reasons and stories behind the ecstatic faces grinning insanely out of the little social media boxes.

Like a lot of cold-water swimmers, my ultimate dream is to sit in an ice hole in the middle of a lake with the sun setting. This is also my nightmare! Imagine having your legs dangling down into the water and how it would feel if something grabbed your feet and pulled you down – I can see my hands now frantically trying to grip on to the icy edge of the hole, my face frozen in a scream of terror!

To face such fears could be the trigger to peeling back the final layers of myself to see what lies right at my core. This could be the way to finally become whole again after all the rebuilding of my physical and emotional strength. But you can't just turn up at a frozen lake, walk out and bash away at thick ice until you have a dark hole big enough to slip into. Definitely a recipe for disaster!

No. I needed to train for this, learn from other people and meet my perfect ice hole with the right amount of knowledge and courage to receive it as the experience I wanted it to be. Along the way, I wanted to discover how other swimmers explained their cold addiction and how it had changed their lives. Had they peeled back their own layers to explore what lay within? Was there an important shared experience within our community and, if so, how could I then translate that into language and imagery relevant to people from beyond the cold-water swimming community? We all push ourselves into 'the zone' when we are doing hard physical things, such as an ultra run, a MTB black run, a duathlon or a sportive, but we all use different mediums to get there.

If I may, I'd like to take a moment to refocus on why I wrote this book and to explain how I went about choosing the right people to help me complete this journey into 'my perfect ice hole' and to explore why I used my 'family' of different characters to sort people into categories.

It started as an idea while driving up to Scotland in my campervan with my son and his girlfriend. I suddenly burst out, 'I know! I know what I need to write about. Quick, can you concentrate for two minutes while I dictate an email?'

And that email was to Vertebrate Publishing, who I thought would be the most receptive publisher for what I wanted to write. Within an hour of sending the email I had my answer: yes, they were potentially interested in discussing the idea further.

The basic premise for my proposal was: what is it about the cold that people love so much?

On a practical note, I wondered how to go about making the idea of sitting in an ice hole a reality. I needed the help of experienced ice bathers and, although we do get good winter conditions here in the UK from time to time, the weather is not reliable. I started to read about the subject and make tentative plans.

Ice bathing and cold-water swimming have both grown exponentially in the UK over recent years, although in parts of northern Europe (in particular Scandinavia) and North America, they are a very real and accepted part of the culture, along with saunas and fairy lights to make the dark days of winter more bearable. Once the ice takes hold and the cold is intense and bitey enough, the stoics emerge. These are some of the people I need to learn from; ice bathing is in their blood. They inhabit lands where the long hours of dark and cold are set on fire with strings of lights and burning coals; fit-for-purpose ladders are lowered into the dark water; ice saws are sharpened ready to cut through thick ice; toasty lakeside saunas are refuelled and crazy landscapes come into their own.

Here in the UK, we are known to be a nation of people who reinvent, recreate and repurpose. If we don't have access to rivers, lakes, waterfalls, the sea or other bodies of water, which may or may not freeze over or at least drop to that holy sub-5° Celsius, we repurpose wheelie bins, chest freezers, galvanised steel troughs and children's paddling pools. And, of course, there is always the cold shower! I can't think of anything worse.

The journey I have been on into colder and colder water has given me the opportunity to go beyond the chaos of physical pain and fear of the future. As I'd peeled back every layer of acquired information, experience and challenge, I had revealed someone I had forgotten existed, someone who I thought I could love and respect. I have always known that I have a force within me. I have referred to it as a 'tiny flame', which I have managed to never let anyone or anything extinguish completely. It has helped me through difficult situations where I needed to be fierce, but not brutal, with myself or with others.

This force is my Warrior, one of the five facets of myself which make up my personality, but each comes into its own at different times. I know that in psychology the term 'archetypes' is used to describe different facets of a person and the number of archetypes can vary wildly from a handful to a hundred or more, but all I know is what I experienced and discussed within those hypnotherapy sessions: the Mother, the Warrior, the Child, the Panther and the Thinker.

To clarify how I see these parts of myself, I can give examples of where I believe I have already used them, even before I had been empowered to name them. On tough, alpine climbs in the Pyrenees or here in the Lake District, I remember zoning out of my body and searching deep down inside myself for the strength and grit I needed to cycle for another twenty kilometres at a gradient of five per cent. Right down through the layers I found my Warrior. That had been the point at which I knew I could reach the summit. I just had to grind my way up, make my focus shift from the burning in my quads to a vision or horizon in my mind that was totally disconnected from where I actually was. It had been almost an out-of-body experience. Physically, I was in such discomfort, so mentally I had to find sanctuary somewhere else until the struggle was over. Alongside this refocus I altered my breathing, so that I could calm the panic flooding through my body, and let my breath take me to another place where I no longer felt as if my insides wanted to burst out of my mouth in a foul spew of pain.

But when I go swimming, it is not this violent. I have never tried to do battle with the cold. It has been my natural inclination to submit and allow everything my body and mind has ever learnt about pain and chaos to take over and protect me. That being said, I have often called on my Warrior to stand by my side while I pluck up the courage to swim out of my depth, work my way across boulders in a stream or scramble down to a beautiful waterfall. On these occasions, I have also noticed the other 'members of my family' come to the fore. For example, if I feel like doing a jetty strut, I know my Panther has come out to play, the side of myself that is in touch with my femininity, my physicality and my sexual energy. When I am planning a walk up to a mountain tarn, I call on my Thinker to make sure I have all I need with me, to check the route and once up at the tarn decide which is the best access and exit point. It takes my Mother sometimes to guide me up the path if I suddenly feel unable to walk any further and need a hand to hold on to. And I reach out my hands to the sky as I launch myself off a jetty into a lake, shrieking with Child-like joy and energy.

I wondered whether other people had similar experiences in their lives, and in particular on their cold-water journeys. Do they call on their Warrior to help them find the courage to immerse in icy cold water? Would it be possible to find people who had similar facets within them to mine? Would we bring out different facets of ourselves when we met?

The more I started to piece together my thinking, the more I realised that I needed to go on a new type of journey, one where I met different cold-water swimmers who all had their own stories to tell about why they loved the cold and how it made them feel.

Initially, I thought I would be able to meet and swim with at least twenty different people from all over the world in their favourite location, whether that be a frozen lake, a wheelie bin, a wooden barrel, a river or the ocean. But there were several practical and logistical issues to work through: how far could I travel on a limited budget and with Covid-19 travel restrictions still in place in many countries; would everyone I asked be willing to talk with me; and how would I go about choosing them in the first place?

The travel was affected by budget and restrictions, but fortunately I was able to work around that using technology such as Zoom video calls, and my campervan acted as a mobile home and office on occasion. I was also amazed by the generosity of several of my interviewees who invited me to stay with them.

A couple of people I contacted changed their minds about being part of the project and a couple of them were also slightly evasive about whether they did or didn't want to be included. I accepted early on that not everyone wants to be in the public eye, especially as seen through someone else's eyes. It did leave me feeling a little disappointed and awkward, especially if I felt I knew the person fairly well already. However, I quickly realised that these negative reactions weren't meant personally, but even so were acting as barriers to the truth. No one is irreplaceable and everyone is entitled to privacy and autonomy. It worked out to be a good frame of mind to adopt, and saved sleepless nights and self-doubt.

When it came to deciding who was a Warrior, Mother, Panther, Child or Thinker, I fell back on social media. The cold-water swimming community I had become part of during the lockdowns is fairly active on social media, which had given me the advantage of observing how people portrayed themselves through photographs, words and interactions. I was already in communication with most of them digitally. From their posts and our interactions it seemed to me that many of them used the cold water as a way to overcome some difficulties and challenges in their lives, so it wasn't a big step from there to wanting to understand what I might find if I peeled back their layers as I had done with my own. Did they believe that the cold water offered the opportunity to go beyond the chaos to find their true selves? Would we be able to peel back those layers together and discover something new about each other?

Out of the sixteen portraits I ended up creating, I actually met ten of the people in real life and not via a video call. It's a good job I'm not risk-averse! Every one of them could have been the wrong 'fit' in the flesh but thankfully, my intuition and observations were pretty accurate. As soon as I started talking to them, it was obvious they fitted the characteristics.

At the beginning of each interview, I explained why I had chosen them, both in terms of the five members of my 'family' and why their swim location intrigued me. Above all else, I wanted to create a portrait of them that was relatable to a broad spectrum of readers. By examining their journey into the cold water and what it meant to them, I hoped to show that wherever you live, whatever your circumstances or budget, there is always a choice in how you can take an ice bath or get in cold water.

One of my more personal reasons for meeting these people was to discover more about myself and how I can feel more complete, how I can finish the journey I started back in February 2017 when I was forced to rethink my whole way of living, to start again, to re-educate my mind and body into a new physicality. I imagined it would be a bit like meeting the different facets of me on a one-to-one basis and seeing what I could take and give within that encounter: shared experiences, similar or different lenses on the world.

A large part of me was apprehensive about meeting total strangers and delving into their lives during an interview and then creating a story about what I had discovered. I felt a huge sense of responsibility towards each and every one of them to get it right, to do them justice and, along the way, even reveal something about them that they didn't know.

The rest of me was excited to travel again, spend time with new people, learn about new things and potentially get a clearer understanding of where and how I wanted to live the next stage of my life now I had turned sixty. The very number felt like a heavy cloud hanging over me. It sounded so old, so useless and powerless. When I was forty I had imagined my life getting better and better; I had not foreseen all the obstacles that have been thrown down in front of me in the intervening years. None of us do.

But I am living that future now and I have to admit, although I have spent long periods feeling unsettled and isolated, I am coming to be more optimistic and curious about what other options I have to my quiet, solitary life in west Cumbria. How can I make full use of the strengths I have within me to reach that place the hypnotherapist said I would be able to find? She said I had all the tools, but I still had no idea how to use them. Maybe other people with similar natures and passions could enlighten me? Maybe we could learn from each other and bring out a different part of each other along the way?

Every day a new article is published about the mental and physical benefits of outdoor swimming and cold-water swimming: boosted immune system, improved blood circulation, reduction to inflammation in joints or nervous system, rejuvenated libido and quelling of menopause symptoms. But that's the science. What about the personal, nonsensical, seemingly inconsequential and quirky reasons? I have plenty of my own highly irrational thoughts as I slip into the cold water, some of which are just too visceral to put into words! But why do other ice bathers crave the cold? What journey have they taken to reach their ice hole, mountain river pool or wheelie bin?

And at the heart of all my thinking was the cold water. It seemed to have released a well of creativity and passion within my soul. What is it about cold water that affects us so intensely? By meeting the Mothers, the Children, the Warriors, the Panthers and the Thinkers from within the cold-water swimming community, I knew I would learn how to better use the tools I already had.

Together, do we hold the key to unlocking the question: what is the cold fix? And how can we use it to live full and happy lives?

THE FELL RUNNER

A bizarre experience in the mountains between a fell runner and me perfectly illustrates how the journey we take in life is moulded by our interactions with people we meet along the way and it reconfirmed why it was so important for me to embark on my journey of meeting a bunch of strangers.

It was one of those Lakeland days when the 'clag' was down and I knew it was going to stay down, but I was on my way to meet a fell runner from the Surrey Hills who was keen to try his hand at wild swimming coupled with a walk up to Scales Tarn. It is actually quite common for me to be contacted by people coming up to the Lakes on holiday and either asked for advice on good places to swim or invited to meet up and swim with them. This guy was a friend of a friend and he had travelled up to the Lakes to support said friend on leg two of the Bob Graham Round.[1]

After a few minutes striding at speed on the first section of the climb up Mousthwaite Comb, he quickly realised, from my heavy breathing and lack of conversation, that I was a mere mortal, not a runner. Fortunately, he turned out to be a bit of a chatterbox, so I didn't need to get many words out as we continued up the steady ascent to where the path met the lower flanks of Scales Fell. No parapents (paragliders) today. It's often a good place to sit and watch them throw themselves off the fell while crossing their fingers they've got the thermals right and they will float over the A66 rather than smear themselves along the white lines.

---

1   The Bob Graham Round, first completed in 1932 by Keswick hotelier Bob Graham, is a sixty-six-mile circuit with 27,000 feet of ascent, linking forty-two of the highest peaks in the English Lake District within twenty-four hours.

We had been trying to guess which fell was Souther Fell and, with my breathing and legs now under control, I was able to join the conversation at last. I love this walk up to Scales Tarn. Even the pull up to this point gets easier the more times you do it, and there's really only one steep bit. Plus, there's a lot to look at from the narrow path that wiggles along below Scales Fell. Most people focus on the craggy, unmistakable outline of Sharp Edge straight ahead, whereas my eyes are scanning the River Glenderamackin in the valley on my right for waterfalls and potential dipping pools.

When we reached the tarn, which was shrouded in mist and low cloud, I guided him round to the left-hand side. A couple of weeks ago I'd been up here with a swim buddy, very early on a gorgeous sunny morning. There was not a breath of wind and the surface of the water was reflecting the surrounding mountains perfectly. We'd been floating about in the middle of the tarn, watching walkers crossing Sharp Edge, a thousand feet straight up above us, when our attention was drawn to a fell runner (a different fell runner!). He had gone round the side of the tarn and was now stripping all his clothes off. With a short skip and stumble he plopped into the tarn and started swimming towards us. 'Good morning,' he said as he swam by. 'Good to see other swimmers up here. I think I can make it to the other side and back before I sink!'

I was glad he had survived because his recommendation of the best entry point now turned out to be accurate. You only had to crawl across one or two rocks, then you were in – up to your eyeballs with twenty metres of crystal-clear, cold water yawning below your feet.

A typical cold-water conversation often deteriorates at this point as the reality of what you are about to do hits you. I knew it was down to me to bring my experience to the fore. I offered to test out the entry point for slipperiness and just as I uttered the fatal words, 'Yeah, I'm not actually slipping … ' – splosh! I fell in awkwardly but without injury.

Time to just settle myself in the cold water and wait for my companion to strip off and join me.

'Got to make sure my cossie doesn't come off,' I heard him laugh from the bank. I turned round automatically and assured him that losing it was the least of his worries.

When a tallish but very skinny man, standing in just his oversized Y-fronts in mizzly rain halfway up a mountain, asks you whether the water he is about to sacrifice himself to is 'tolerable', just what are you supposed to say?

'I don't know,' I answered. 'You might find it horrible. It's cold for me, I have to say!'

'Righto. That could be a bit of a problem, then.' But his voice was still cheerful.

I was feeling fine. I was sitting in the tarn up to my armpits, but as I watched his bare feet treading carefully across the stones, I looked up and clocked the intense concentration on his face. I melted and held out my hand. 'Just come and sit here. Take my hand if you want.'

He brushed it away. 'It's alright. It's not slippery.'

He was almost at my side, doing really well, still able to talk, but struggling with his breath. The last thing I wanted him to do was slip: fall into the water, inhale a huge mouthful of water and we'd suddenly be in trouble. 'Focus on your breathing,' I told him.

Loud inhales and exhales and lots of aaaahhhs.

'Just breathe,' I repeated.

'Aaaaaahhh, aaaaaaaaahhh. Balance,' he reminded himself.

'Just balance your mind and your body.' Then I thought of something that might help him, 'You know when you're on a horrible bit of a fell race?'

No answer. From that point on, the only sounds uttered by my 'pupil' were weird laughs, rightos, eeeeees, aaaaaahs and baaaas, or so it seemed. There were also a few sheep watching us!

'In through your nose and out through your mouth. That's it.' I looked back at the bank and laughed. 'Hah! Your backside is on camera. So, you're going to have to get in the water.'

This stranger laughed, but had come to a frozen standstill. He was half crouched, half squatting in the tarn.

'Here, hold my hand, honestly ... ' I urged him. He took it and gripped really hard. 'Right, yes, that's it, strong, big deep breath. In through your nose and out through your mouth ... hmmm, that'll be the hardest bit,' I added as I saw him jiggling up and down, trying to dip his nether regions in daintily with the minimum of pain.

Eeeeeeee, eeeeeeeee, eeeeeeeeeee and lots of heavy breathing echoed round the mist-filled cirque tarn.

I couldn't resist. 'You sound like you're having a baby!' Cruel, I know, but … 'You're doing really well,' I added, wishing he'd not grip my hand quite so hard; it was turning blue. 'Keep going. Here, my other hand will feel warm.' I reached across and wrapped my right hand over both of his, just to remind him that there was something cosy about the day.

'Can you get right down? Do you want to let go and balance yourself?' I heard myself talking extra slowly, as if he was a foreigner who didn't have a clear grasp of English.

He tried releasing my hand and lowering himself a little further, but quickly grabbed at me again, without uttering a word, just staring at me with huge blue eyes as if begging for this to stop. It was an intense moment.

My eyes locked on to his and I repeated, 'In through your nose and out through your mouth and focus there, over there into the mist. The pain's just … '

'Don't think … just swim … ' The first fully formed first words he'd managed since he'd squatted at my side.

'You don't think you can swim? Right, down a bit more. Sit.'

'I can walk,' he grunted.

'Don't swim out of your depth until you've got yourself under control. Okay? And if you want to get out, get out!' I smiled at him, relenting a little. 'It is cold.'

'Yeah … Righto, I think that's me … ' And he stood up, let go of my hand and made his way out of the water as fast as he could without falling.

'Right, don't slip getting out. Go on, I'm going to have a quick little swim once I know you're out safely. Grab my microfibre thing if you want and get dressed. Have a hot drink. I'm not being bossy, I'm just … '

But he didn't seem in the slightest bit bothered about having been told what to do. 'Golly, at least I got my crotch in,' he laughed from under the microfibre changing robe, which he'd got on back to front.

As I swam out into the mist I could hear him chuckling away to himself as he dried off. I longed just to keep swimming and be lost in grey drizzle.

'It's hard to know whether in terms of like, okay, the compliment …

in this situation it's a compliment for me to say you have more insulation than me,' his voice carried across the water.

It's true. I am not overweight, but I do carry a reasonable insulating layer of body fat all over, but in particular around my middle. He's right, on occasions like this, being skinny as a whippet, with zero insulation, is not helpful. As he put it, 'It's like attacking the organs straight away and the circulation.'

Briefly, I zoned out, acutely aware of how beautiful the water felt through my fingers, the chill of the deep aqua below me and the intoxicating scent of Lakeland clag coating my hair. Heaven.

His voice broke into my trance. 'I tell you also why I'm a bit wussy, it's because, you know, a history of heart attack, like with my father.'

'Oh God!' I turned round immediately and swam back to shore. A reality check.

'Yeah, so I just don't know what the ... when it's cold, that was the coldest water I've ever been in swimming, so you just don't know.' He was scaring me silly. Why hadn't he mentioned heart attacks in the family before?

'When you're being induced ... what's the right word, is it an induction? Um, what's the right word when you're introduced to something?'

'Baptism ... ' I started to say, but he carried on his train of thought.

'Enunciation?'

'I don't know ... baptism by fire?' I said, now perched on a slimy rock.

'Ha ha, baptism by frozen balls more like, ha ha.' He was on such a high, which was wonderful to see. I was also glad that he had got himself dressed with no side effects, other than hysterical laughing.

He continued, 'This sounds to me quite like the Buddhist, you know, the Buddhist kind of like thrashing themselves with sticks ... hah, the same sort of thing?'

'I suppose it is a bit.' I was picking my way carefully out of the water now. The stones felt uncomfortable, but I wasn't at all cold.

'You have to have some sort of ... degree ... of suffering. It is a sense of redemption. So, it seems to me, is it, there's an aspect here, you know, secular religious substitute, where you're in a purification process ... um, going through pain, um ... '

Well, there was clearly nothing wrong with his mental faculties after his initiation into cold water! But he had a point. It was a fascinating concept that hadn't crossed my mind before in the context of cold-water swimming.

'You can say the same about fell running,' he continued. 'A sort of test in the wilderness sort of thing … '

That was exactly why I had told him to imagine himself 'on a horrible bit of a fell race', such as a technically difficult section of the Bob Graham, which required him to dig deep. To dig into a different part of his brain. The one that was primordial, to do with survival, not rational thinking.

We finished our swim with hot tea and cake, which tasted delicious, especially because we were both on the verge of shivering. I know my body burns way more energy in cold water, just to keep everything warm. This tall, skinny man then took my hand and said we should hold hands for a bit to cement the bond we had created by holding hands in the water.

Trust. Imagine the trust this guy must have placed in me. We'd never met before and only exchanged a few messages to arrange this meetup. But I had seen it in his eyes, felt it in his grip and now it overwhelmed us both as we sat staring out at the masterpiece that lay before us: furls of mist clinging to the surface of Scales Tarn.

This extraordinary level of trust and meeting of minds is at the core of the cold-water and ice-bathing community. We are all individuals with our quirks and qualities, but we also have similarities and shared experiences. There seems to be a common desire to encourage and nurture, to champion and protect, to play and be curious, to celebrate our bodies and the physical, even sensual qualities of the cold, to question the 'norm' and reflect on how we want to live our lives.

I had been the Mother to his Child, the Warrior to his Thinker, but neither of our Panthers had had an interest in coming out to play, thank goodness!

MEETING
STRANGERS

THE
MOTHER

Non-judgemental, nurturing, a provider of nourishment for the
body and emotions, tactile and physical, healthy and strong,
natural inner and outer beauty, fertile energy and creativity.

CLAUDIA

Claudia is about my age and divides her time between St-Jean-Cap-Ferrat on the Mediterranean coast and St-André-les-Alpes in the Alpes-de-Haute-Provence. She's a self-confessed swimsuit and wool junkie, both of which she needs on a daily basis. She's German by birth, but living in France most of her life has given Claudia the best of both worlds in many ways.

I'm not sure we stopped talking from the moment she burst in through her apartment's glass and ironwork front door to the moment she hugged me goodbye at the security gate in Nice Airport. Three days of sharing our life stories, laughing and crying together about motherhood, relationships and growing older. Writing this now, I am struck by how much I miss Claudia's energy and very practical and direct approach to life.

It had felt weird to be travelling abroad again – so many hurdles to overcome: packing everything I thought I needed into a small cabin bag; all the Covid paperwork; adaptor plugs; and worrying about the height of Gloria, my VW campervan. So, I broke the fear down into small steps: drive south on the M6, which intimidated me after months of negotiating small, statistically more lethal, rural roads in the Lake District; check into the Premier Inn near Manchester Airport; not sleep through the alarm at 5.15; tea and porridge in bed, then shower. All good so far, but then the barrier wouldn't open at the mid-stay car park. I pressed various buttons, but nothing moved, only my guts. The lady in the barrier machine had no record of a booking. I stared blankly at my paperwork trying to work out why not, acutely aware this could all go horribly wrong. The dates on the email … shit! I had booked the wrong dates because I'd changed from multi-storey to mid-stay and back several times because of the height restrictions.

But, fortunately, an angel must have been hovering around the barrier machine, impatient to see me off on my journey. Sue, the lady in the machine, weirdly decided that as I was a 'frequent visitor' to Manchester Airport (I wasn't going to argue!) she would allow me in.

My sense of panic sat like solid porridge at the back of my throat, but I held it down, just. A little song of joy played softly somewhere in my brain, threading its way to the tips of my fingers and toes. I was getting there. The adventure was beginning. Here I was, escaping a Cumbrian November for the Mediterranean, going back to somewhere a part of me has always belonged: France.

Franz, Claudia's son, stood in the arrivals hall at Nice Airport, staring at everyone who looked remotely like a swimmer. My salt and mud-stained jeans and T-shirt (from squeezing past Gloria in the car park) must have spoken to him because he immediately lowered his shades, smiled and walked towards me. Claudia was still at work in Monaco, so she'd asked Franz to meet me off the flight and look after me until she got home.

It felt good to be on the wrong side of the car on the right side of the road, drifting along the Promenade des Anglais next to the azure sea, finishing off my airport-bought salami baguette. The last time I had been there was when I was a student and doing my third year in France as a French assistant and I had spent the last six weeks or so sharing an apartment in old Nice with some English girls. We spent a lot of time on the beach, learning French from the locals, which included balancing on the back of a two-stroke motorbike while the driver negotiated the narrow, cobbled streets and surprise corners.

Cap-Ferrat is a mix of secluded, coast-hugging mini chateaux and apartment blocks, its narrow streets lined with cafes, bars, boulangeries, charcuteries and épiceries. Claudia's apartment is an eclectic mix of plants, photographs, paintings and millions of balls and skeins of wool, and has stunning views in all directions across terracotta rooftops. While we were waiting for his mother to return from work, Franz offered to show me their local beach, Beaulieu. It was a blissful 18 °C in the clear sea. What cold fix? Why did I need a cold fix when I could have this holistic warm bath?

My first sunrise swim with Claudia lay at the end of a footpath that wound close to the edge of Cap-Ferrat, past iconic palm trees, mock palaces not dissimilar to the pink palace of nearby Monte Carlo, storm-battered private jetties and early morning joggers and dog walkers.

Using a building-site fence as a clothes line, we stripped down to swim-suits in the cool air. I shivered. It was a quiet, misty morning, with hardly any sign of the sun, but I was excited to be in the water with Claudia. How far did she swim? Did she swim breaststroke? Would I be able to keep up with her? And then I fell silent. On the horizon something beautiful was happening, subtle but mesmerising. I wanted to get out of my mind and into my body, into the moment.

After about twenty minutes, even at 17 °C, the water began to feel cold and we either needed to swim properly or get out, but I persuaded Claudia to do something she told me she never normally does: get her head wet. I taught her how to do a hair flick on the condition that straight afterwards we'd walk to the nearest boulangerie, which sold not only delicious croissants but piping-hot takeaway espressos.

During lockdown people had been forbidden to go on to the beach, so instead Claudia had recommissioned her children's 150-centimetre plastic paddling pool. After her early morning permitted walk within a kilometre of home, her roof terrace was where she bathed, in water only thirty-five centimetres deep, but often just 4 °C.

Her first experience with sub-5° water had been in March 2019, visiting her brother and his family in Finland. Her sister-in-law took her to dip in the Baltic Sea, where the water was 4 °C, the air temperature -14 °C. The sea was frozen, apart from a small hole at the foot of the ladder near the purpose-built hut where you changed and warmed up post-dip. As she peered down into the hole, a few blocks of ice floated across it. But a voice in her head stopped her from running away: 'How hard can it be? If others can do it, so can I.' As she climbed down the ladder and into the water, nothing changed, but with the first movement in the slush she gasped and breathing was difficult. She scrambled back up the ladder immediately. Not to be beaten, she returned the next day and the next, staying in a few seconds longer each time. She hadn't expected the initial feeling to be so intense, so had paid no attention to her breathing. A week of bathing daily and focusing on breathing calmly as she entered the water got her hooked, but there was not another opportunity to ice bathe, partly due to lockdown and travel restrictions. Instead, in her tiny, roof-terrace ice bath she taught herself to breathe and accept the cold.[2]

Sometimes, as she lay there, her mind went on journeys, back in time. To Germany and her grandfather, Opa Franz, a very special person with whom she had lived between the ages of six and seven. Every day between May and September, she shared his daily routine. He would wake her at dawn and, dressed only in bathrobes, no shoes, they would drive to the outdoor pool set in the nearby forest and swim for half an hour in cool water. The feel of frosted grass under her bare feet is synonymous with that time, along with the smell of the bakery where they stopped on the way home to buy bread for breakfast. She never gave the cold a thought – it was just what they did, and it held no fear for her.

Once allowed to travel to the mountains again, and her home in St André-les-Alpes, she sought out the river, wondering whether her paddling-pool experience would have changed her relationship to the fast-flowing cold water. At first, her natural aversion to risk almost held her back, but as familiarity with the river and its safe spots grew, so did her bravery, until one snowy day, when the air temperature was a toe-tingling -12 °C and the water 1 °C, she realised a personal dream. In a landscape designed to be photographed – blue sky, white snow and black skeletal trees set against snow-capped mountains – she officially broke ice and created her own pocket of cold heaven. With her husband hovering around anxiously, Claudia cleared away enough ice to create a little space, and this act of preparation helped to calm her excitement. She felt no fear, just anticipation at what she was about to experience.

'Ice around me feels like a protective layer. Most people in my life don't like cold water, so when I go into the water nobody can reach me. I can swim away from all pressure and stress until I feel ready to return.'

2   Claudia wanted me to share the temperatures of her different swim spots: Mediterranean (min. winter 12 °C, max. summer 26 °C), Lac de Castillon (min. winter 6 °C, max. summer 24 °C), River Verdon (min. winter 1 °C, max. summer 17 °C), Baltic Sea in Hanko, Finland (min. winter 1 °C, max. summer 27 °C).

For such an active woman, Claudia deliberately seeks out these moments of stillness in the river because it is only within them that she finds peace. First, she walks fast for an hour, her mind fizzing and buzzing with everything from new ideas for knitting creations to recipes for what to eat for dinner and solutions to difficult situations with family or work. Entering the water immediately clears her mind; the colder the water, the quicker she stops thinking. Nothing else matters except nature around her, the noise of the water, the air, the birds and watching bubbles in the river.

We had hurried to this same river from the train station in St-André-les-Alpes on the day after I arrived at Claudia's. We'd caught the lunchtime train from Nice, which chugged its way up from the coast into the Alpes-de-Haute-Provence, knowing that we would only have time to dump our bags on the terrace of the mountain home she shared with her husband before racing against the sun as it slipped away behind the mountains. A slight mist hovered above the fast-flowing river. I shivered slightly as I stood in my swimsuit watching Claudia set up her phone inside one of her boots. Finding our balance on the grey, water-rounded stones had us waving our arms about like helicopters, shrieking, our legs stretched from one secure foothold to another, praying we would suddenly become graceful creatures. And then, like disgruntled children, we plonked ourselves down in two separate eddies, squealing at the bite of the cold water and laughing out loud at each other.

And then came the solitary, but shared, quiet contemplation. For me, every second of this experience meant so much; I didn't want it to end. For Claudia, it was her weekend ritual, so would only end if she didn't live there any more. Bittersweet thoughts battled in my head and I couldn't find any peace from them. I longed to live here, but I wanted the people I care about to be here with me.

I completely understood why, whatever the weather, she comes here at sunrise each day: soaking up the natural beauty of the landscape is her main motivation; the cold is a close second. And in the winter months she has it all to herself. Nothing else comes close to giving her what this gives her.

Not even the turquoise Lac de Castillon where, the following lunchtime, we met up with some of her friends and swam together. Set north of the iconic Gorges du Verdon, this is actually a reservoir, but one where watersports, including swimming, are permitted. We were a noisy, chatty group of men and women as we walked from the cars to the lakeshore to change. The conversation revolved around food and whether or not I would be allowed to film underwater because Jean-Luc might leave a trail of bubbles behind him as he swam. Or at least that's what I thought he was worried about. My university French is good and I was just about holding my own in the fast-moving conversations around me, but you just never know if you have correctly translated the humour or not!

Claudia had encouraged friends from St-André to swim here every Saturday lunchtime after the traditional trip to the local market and hoped this would be the first winter they would keep swimming as the temperatures dropped. Her only concern was that none of them seemed to feel the cold, so she sometimes had to tell them to get out. She'd encouraged them to take a hot drink, to swim less distance, stay in for less time, even just walk on the spot in the water, but at least to keep the routine going. Some of them were even talking of buying swim robes and neoprene gloves, so it seemed her motivational spirit was winning them over.

The lake is a midway point between the sea and the river in terms of temperature and activity. Here, Claudia can actually swim for at least twenty minutes, because the water rarely drops below 6 °C, so it becomes more of a moving meditation for her. Once, when her husband was away, she swam right out into the middle of the lake and didn't want to stop. So, she just kept swimming, to the other side and back.

'All mine.' Those were her words to describe how that adventure had made her feel. Out there she had only had responsibility for herself. In the water, people couldn't reach her emotionally and psychologically. She knows that every time she comes out of the water she will be a different person to the one who went in. She has regained control over her own life because in the water it is down to her to decide when to come out. In winter, on a cold day, she feels out of contact and yet in total contact with her sense of self.

On our last evening, we returned by train to her St-Jean apartment. It was as if by inviting me into her mountain space, something had shifted deep within Claudia, because while we were talking quietly over our final glass of Prosecco, she started to cry silently. She seemed to shrink away from the world into her sofa, in the same way that she retreats from the world into the water. This vibrant, gorgeous woman with whom I had spent nearly three days talking non-stop had turned inside out. My heart went out to her. I paused the voice recorder and reached over to hold her in my arms.

Claudia's way through recent difficult moments with family members had been the cold water. Lying in the river, in particular, had allowed her to distance herself enough from the situation to be able to think clearly about how she could help, what words she could use that wouldn't act as triggers. Her practical nature could see that in order to get perspective she had to remove herself from the middle of the problem; in a way she had to step outside her own head and heart and become a stranger to the issue.

But I was left with the nagging feeling that before meeting Claudia I had automatically put her in the Mother character category because that's how I saw her. But was she? Or had she, by opening up to me, become more of the Child and me the Mother? Human relationships and interactions are so complex and if we all have these different characters within us, then of course it is natural that we each bring out different qualities in each other. I think this is going to be a far more complicated journey than I had originally anticipated!

SOLVEIG

Solveig is sixty-seven years old. She lives with her husband in southern Norway. She started swimming in 2007, so this is her fourteenth winter. At first she swam every week, and then on 25 May 2020 she started to swim every day.

I came to Solveig's tiny Airbnb on a cold, dark December night, not sure who I was meeting or where I was staying. She and her husband had fetched me from another swimmer's house and introduced me to my first Norwegian supermarket en route to their home on the island of Hisøy, near Arendal, in Norway's 'Riviera'.

Left on my own to unpack and settle in while they prepared dinner up in their own house, I was suddenly overwhelmed by what I had undertaken. I felt lost and frightened, in spite of the enormous generosity and warmth of my hosts so far. I felt a huge weight of responsibility to somehow return the favour and had no idea how. Money hadn't exchanged hands, and, although I had brought each of them a small gift from the Lake District, I felt as if I was giving them nothing back. They were investing emotionally in me and I had no idea whether I could deliver. The time we spent together wasn't set in stone; there was no agenda other than to make some sort of connection through our shared passion for cold water. I'm not sure I have ever put myself in such a strange situation in my life, staying in the homes of strangers and just going with the flow! Is this the magic of the cold-water swimming community? Do we really have a connection that runs deeper than other communities of like-minded people? Or have I just struck lucky with my choice of hosts so far?

After a delicious dinner, Solveig and I walked side by side, each holding on to an antique sledge with one hand and a lantern with the other. The sledge was to give us some sort of balance on the icy track that led down from her house to the beach. Gritting and salting roads in Norway is almost unheard of. People and cars endure treacherous conditions for months on end, relying on balance, grippers, and the winter or studded tyres that are mandatory on their vehicles. Solveig wears heavy boots and seems to have perfected a way of half walking, half skating everywhere she goes. My own winter boots have inbuilt spikes that can be folded out using a tiny tool or, on special occasions, a teaspoon. Solveig told me about another time when she was going so fast with the sledge that it ran away with her. She had fallen on to her knees and was still holding on to the handlebars. But after struggling up again she had kept going down to the beach, undressed and walked straight into the sea. Miraculously, there was no pain or bruising from her fall. And then she told me she has osteoporosis!

I squinted by the gleam of my bobble hat full of fairy lights in amazement at this vibrant Norwegian lady next to me, dressed in many layers of woollen clothes, including a long red skirt made from fabric bought over fifty years ago when she and a friend, aged twelve, had taken the bus to Kristiansand, with the sole aim of visiting a store that made the Norwegian national costume. The fabric is harsh and thin, but so closely woven that it stops the wind. From 1 December until the first day of spring, she wears it to go to the beach: a small but precious memory, red like the lipstick she always wears, even when swimming. Solveig's complicated life overwhelms her sometimes, but the skirt, the lipstick and the swimming all remind her that beneath her worries and stresses there is a strong foundation of love and faith.

That night we swam together, just the two of us, but she loves the feel of community she experiences with the groups she has built up; swimming with her mermaids and mermen makes her laugh and she desperately wants laughter in her life. Sometimes she wonders what they think of her, what an 'old lady' like her can give them. But most of the time she feels strong and ageless; the new and familiar people she meets each day in the water are her cold-water family. The conversations in the water continue on dry land while they are changing. It feels as if she has something that is just hers again, like when she was a child. For so many years she has given, to family, to her four jobs.

It was in between her work and family commitments that I met up with Solveig again the following day for a group swim. It was one of her 'down under' days and I knew I would be going 'down under' with her whether I liked it or not! Fortunately, I love full immersion, even in cold water, so dunking down, or duck diving, is definitely a big part of my dips or swims. I feel far more alive if I've got wet all over. But Solveig's description took it to another level: 'Going down under the water is like being in my bed; it feels like a blanket around me.'

At first she feels a pain at the back of her neck, and if it keeps hurting she keeps her head higher up and waits a few seconds for the cold to sink in. It can feel like a nail driving into the back of her neck. She breathes the water in and sits on the bottom. The water is right up in her sinuses, but then as she surfaces she blows it out hard from inside her head. She is not afraid of being under the water and taking the water in. Believe me, I've seen her do it and it definitely takes her three dunks! Then she is done.

One of Solveig's other habits is to gesticulate – a lot. 'Oh yes, I speak with my hands, so the pandemic changed my life. I used to get close to people to show them I care; I would use my hands to make sure you had everything you needed. When I hug you it is because I want to make sure you're okay. When I'm under the water it is as if I am being hugged. I hold out my hands and want someone to take hold of them. My hands are my strongest way of communicating how I feel. I want to be that person again.'

I had noticed that all the ladies I swam with on Solveig's beach wore thick, oiled wool mittens and kept their hands out of the water. It is almost as if they were holding their hands up in surrender – to the cold water maybe? But I couldn't imagine Solveig ever surrendering to anything or anyone. 'But I do, I let the cold water take the physical pain of osteoarthritis away from my body.'

It wasn't icy in the sea when I was there, although there was plenty of snow on the beach and I wondered how Solveig felt about ice: did she just walk into a frozen or slushy sea, or did she prepare herself first, with some breathwork or exercises? Her face lit up and she threw her hands up in the air, waving wildly: this, I imagine, was how she greeted the arrival of ice!

'It was amazing last winter,' she says. 'We had so much ice and it lasted for so long. We had to use an axe here in the sea, but we had no axe. I found a piece of wood which had washed up and I prepared an ice-free entry point for the other swimmers. The ice gave me cuts, but I was so excited to get in. I should have been more careful as I have varicose veins so I would bleed badly if I am cut too deeply.'

Her laughter is a full-body experience and completely out of sync with the seriousness of what she was talking about. But I understood why. One of the first things Solveig said to me was, 'I like to be a mum, look after my kids, my husband, to make food, to nurse and take care of people, and I have always wanted to be responsible for my own life and bring my kids up to feel the same.' All of that caring for other people takes its toll even on someone who seems to have limitless capacity for giving. The swift transition from serious to joy is what Solveig seeks on a daily basis. Even in the short space of a couple of days spent together, I witnessed Solveig exhausted and drained from commitment to others and then become rejuvenated almost as soon as her toes touched the water. I watched the cold burst the heavy cloud and bring immediate relief.

LEELOU

Leelou has lived in the South Lakes virtually all her life and has worked within the caring profession in one capacity or another for what probably seems like forever, but loves it. In her current role she works with elderly clients to ensure they are able to lead as independent a life as possible. Time off is spent with family and friends, swimming, cooking, walking and thinking about food.

'I used to buy ice creams from there when I was a little girl.' Leelou pointed at the barn end of the farmhouse down at Millerground on Lake Windermere. 'And, look! Why've I never noticed that on top of it before?' We both stopped on the trudge back up the track to our cars and I looked to where she was pointing. An arch, as if there should be a bell suspended from it to ring out on Sunday mornings and in times of warning. Stone-built, dramatic and unnoticed by Leelou for nearly fifty years of coming to this place.

'I look up more these days,' she said, when in fact the opposite is almost always true of people as they grow older, for fear of tripping! Or is that just me?

But one thing I had noticed about Leelou every time we'd swum together is how observant she is of what is around her: from the taste and quality of the water she's immersed in, to the play of the light on the fells and trees. It's so much more striking in winter when you can see right through stands of skeletal trees; your depth of focus is greater and the light somehow more transparent. Do we become more aware of our surroundings when electronic distractions and white noise disappear? Or is it connected to the temperature of the water? As the temperature drops, self-awareness increases? As the blood rushes to our core to keep our vital organs safe, is something switched on in our brains that reconnects us to all our senses?

I watched Leelou's face as she sank down slowly and luxuriantly into the lake on a grey-tinged-pink January morning; my intrusion into her unguarded emotions felt connecting and completing. I was her and she was me. My facial muscles tensed and relaxed in a similar way every time I submitted to the cold. We were in this together, in that one moment of change. Silence. Except for a wagtail on the jetty, two seagulls squawking in harmony below a cloud, we didn't even make a ripple on the surface of the lake; our strokes were so slow and almost meditative.

Once we had settled into the temperature, we began to talk while our bodies automatically pulled and worked through the water, as if they were trained to take those precious strokes repeatedly until our brains bid them stop. This is the only place I can successfully multi-task, here in a calm, silent lake. I could swim before I could walk, so my entire body is familiar with being in water and staying afloat.

As we swam back and forth between the jetties, Leelou and I mused over how the cold water has become intrinsically woven into our daily life. During lockdown, the swimming pools were closed, so like many dedicated indoor swimmers Leelou had become very frustrated. Her husband bore the brunt of her stir-craziness and kept suggesting she try swimming outdoors, a thought that horrified her because she knew there were fish in Lake Windermere. But eventually, for her husband's sake, she agreed to give it a try.

When she first hit the water she got the most amazing feeling – it was early May, so the water temperature was still only around 12 °C. It was as if her skin was on fire from the touch of the water and she felt euphoric. So she continued to swim solo while her husband stayed close by on the bank.

One magic moment she will never forget, because it transformed her fear of the water into love, was a late-night swim in Windermere, solo, but with her husband as spotter. It was about 9.45 p.m. in summer, so still light. She swam on her own from the jetty to the buoy, about 400 metres there and back, slowly, trying not to make any ripples in the water because the surface looked far too beautiful to spoil, like glass. Then something touched her leg. Of course, it made her jump a little, but then she calmed herself by saying over and over, 'I'm just water, at one with the water. I am a part of this water, I belong here.'

This sense of belonging intensified when two ladies from the local mental health swims encouraged her to try the Polar Bear Challenge in 2020–21 (this is a winter swimming challenge that starts at the beginning of November and ends on the last day of March and requires the swimmer to wear no neoprene. There are several levels within the challenge; the basic one is 200 metres twice a month). They promised to support her and swim with her. At first she was nervous about going through her first winter, but found that the colder the water got, the more excited she felt both before and after the swim. The odd thing was that she found there was a feeling of warmth about the water, not from the thrill of it, but just from inside her own body. At home, she rarely switches the heating on, because she finds it far too hot. The feeling she got from the water was different from the occasional hot flushes from the menopause and all she can say is that nothing had ever felt like this before.

Most people rush to get dry and dressed after a swim, but Leelou has never felt cold, preferring to stand around in her swimsuit afterwards with no sense of urgency. She calls it 'air drying' and it is part of the process of allowing the cold water to bring her entire body and being back down to a normal level physically.

Calm, tingle, relaxed, flow. These are some of the words I heard her use while we were talking. Everything about the experience is a positive. Her breath feels good; even the breathless feeling at the first point of immersion is a good feeling. It resets her. It is often the only time she can actually feel the cold and it doesn't last long, but then changes to simply feeling good.

For most of her adult life, like many people, she has suffered from seasonal sadness quite badly and although she loves the seasons, she had come to accept that winter was a dark and difficult time for her. It didn't make her depressed, but just left her with low mood and activity levels. Since starting to swim every day, she no longer feels like this about the change of seasons. In the autumn she has a sense of excitement and anticipation about the difference in temperature, even for rain, wind and snow – and she now can even contemplate those days that never seem to get light with a certain eagerness.

For her, food has always been a big motivator and driver. Now she swims daily, it is even more so, because she feels less self-conscious about her body shape and gives herself the pleasure of looking forward to eating something tasty after her swim. The preparation of good food to make people happy gives her enormous pleasure.

And it is into the water that she takes her physical pain, every day if possible, because if she misses a day her body will soon let her know by aching or sharp pains. She has been known to take her swimsuit to work and stand outside in the rain in it for the sheer relief it gives her.

'This is my fix,' said Leelou. 'To be hugged and held so lightly and yet so deeply. No pain, no need to hug back or ask for more. As soon as I sink down, I feel held close, comforted and all pain is released into the water. My body feels light and happy. I don't need to swim, just be in the cold water.'

I wondered if this overwhelming desire to be hugged by the cold becomes stronger the more you give of yourself in other aspects of your life. Leelou's work involves managing other people's needs, ensuring they continue to lead fulfilling lives as they grow older. And she is a mother, daughter and wife.

'I am not afraid of the cold,' said Leelou. Which didn't answer my question, but led to another line of conversation, about roots. Where do you feel rooted, and does it help to be in familiar surroundings as you make the transition from the comfortable – swimming pools and summer dipping – to the uncomfortable environment of winter swimming? The River Sprint at Sprint Mill, in a remote valley in the South-East Lake District, is where she would consider her roots to be, but she now sees it with fresh eyes: there are places, special places, to explore and get lost in nature. Tiny waterfalls and river pools, visited only by skylarks and sheep, but a treasure trove of dipping spots throughout the year. As a girl she loved it for its familiarity and sense of home, but only 'found' the beauty of the water in adulthood.

'It gives me the best hugs, perhaps because we know each other so well.'

The landscape is like a Mother to Leelou – it loves her unconditionally. Do I feel a connection with Leelou because I miss my mum? Is this why I have felt so strongly about these three women I have called 'Mother'? Or do they bring out the Mother in me? All three could be Warriors too in their own way – the solid support and steadfast fierceness. But above all, I feel in some way very safe with each of them. I suppose I am lucky in that I had a good relationship with my own mother, most of the time. Maybe we were too close at times. But I know she loved me; she protected me right up until the end.

THE
WARRIOR

My Warrior is an enigmatic, calm, strong presence who is
always by my side, ready to be fierce and protect me, or quiet
and watch over me. Neither male nor female. No definable age,
ethnicity or origin.

RYAN

After spending most of his life using linear thinking and numbing himself with stimulants to avoid his feelings, Ryan now embraces the whole of life with both hands. Personal challenges and developments have given him the ability to find and offer a deep presence to others.

Through life experience, learning and practice, he has developed a profound understanding of and empathy for the human condition. He has acquired skills and tools which he shares with others so they can have them at their disposal whenever they desire reconnection or situations become challenging. These skills include functional breathwork, ice therapy, coaching, meditation and embodiment.

Ryan's mission is to build a community by helping others optimise their human experience and let go of their own limiting beliefs, so they can fully embrace themselves in the here and now.

Cold for Ryan is a metaphor for the chaos of life: rushing out of the door in the morning, extreme weather patterns, interactions with other people in our lives or with strangers. There is a flow of chaos in life that we have the opportunity to resist or allow, but when we allow it to run through us, it can make life much more enjoyable. We can also train ourselves to deal with stress and chaos, to build our resistance to it in the same way that we can do resistance training for our muscles. An ice bath, or extreme cold, is one opportunity to build resilience by stepping into the chaos or stressful environment.

'I believe that to optimise that experience it is important to soften into it, to have the ability to create space in the body and mind in the middle of it.' Ryan recognises the amazing biological effects achieved just by regular cold-water immersion, but what he is looking for goes beyond that. If we want to change thought and behaviour patterns, we need to create that little bit of space between 'reacting' and 'responding'.

'You know how you gasp when you first get in cold water? This reaction is the same as when your partner forgets to put out the bin and you snap at them. There is no space between their action and your reaction, but if you train yourself to take even just one small breath, you are already creating enough space on a biological and spiritual level to retread the path.'

This type of self-regulation can control the parasympathetic environment and eventually bring about change in thought patterns and behaviour because you're repeatedly telling your nervous system a different story.

Ryan's own story started about ten years ago when he went through a series of challenging circumstances: he lost his dad to cancer after having cared for him, fractured his spine and herniated a disc in an accident, gave up his job to become self-employed, became a father and struggled with the impact of his son's diagnosis of cystic fibrosis and had relationship struggles.

He tried to deal with all of this on his own by pushing through the week and not paying attention to his alcohol intake or general health. The situation couldn't continue. Ryan desperately wanted to find a way to change and heal himself. Then his path crossed with that of a woman called Sue, who was a yogi.

She taught him Dru yoga, which is a sequence of movements that can become a powerful practice for the body and mind. Not only does it release fascia in the body, but it gave him permission to respond to life's challenges with kindness to himself and others. If only he had met her while he was caring for his dad during his last weeks of life, the impact of constantly trying to calm his dad's nervous system might not have been so unbelievably hard. The only thing that had enabled him to keep strong was the belief that the deeper into the dark you go, the further into the light you step.

The final piece in the jigsaw was when Ryan moved from mouth breathing to nose breathing during a conscious creative breath workshop he attended. He had noticed that mouth breathing and Wim-Hof-type breathwork had increased his anxiety, but as soon as he switched to nose breathing, his entire parasympathetic nervous system calmed down. Combined with an ice bath, he had all the information he needed.

'The cold became my anchor,' said Ryan. And once he had that anchor, he felt able to teach others.

He started with a barrel in his back garden to train in cold water for an upcoming triathlon. The challenge for him wasn't the running, cycling or swimming; it was to do everything by breathing through his nose. But daily immersion in his ice barrel triggered an enjoyment for endurance training he didn't realise he needed. He started to feel really good and looked better. The final wall he had to break down was his inability to talk in a group setting and if he was going to work with groups of people, he knew this would hold him back. Instead of backing away, he leant into this resistance and started to post about his journey on social media. He felt physically sick, but kept leaning into it.

Wind forward to a sunny autumnal day and I was attending a one-to-one workshop at Ryan's studio.

The first session of the day was a gentle, silent walk through the woods behind Ryan's property. I am a natural nose breather, which may have helped me get into this activity more easily. But I haven't ever examined the benefits of this type of breathing, or tried to control my inward and outward breaths while walking. At first, I felt light-headed and didn't enjoy holding my breath while still moving: it felt counterintuitive and I desperately wanted to open my mouth. I was hungry for air, but persevered.

We walked at our own pace, mostly in silence, for around an hour, taking note of how our breathing felt and how we needed to adjust our pace to prolong the breath-holding more comfortably. I soon realised that I wasn't going to actually pass out or be sick, which gave me the confidence to play around with my own breath and movements. My senses tuned in more deeply to my surroundings, in particular sight and sound. I heard every crack of twig under my light step and caught shadows and sunbeams on the periphery of my gaze. My nasal passages felt alive and sensitive to temperature and scent: the deeper woodland areas exuded fungi and damp bark, cool mounds of leaves and warmer hues of fresh-fallen conkers.

All too soon we emerged into a pasture which was surrounded by a tall, barbed-wire fence. It was almost as if the gentle green grass was the transition between our nature bathing and the real world of No Trespassing signs and security guards. A brutal shift between two approaches to life. But, just before leaving our state of relaxation, I realised there had been a deep sense of movement somewhere down inside me, as if chinks of light had opened up in my being, purely through the work of my breath.

I was excited to explore the power of breathing further in our next session, which Ryan explained was an opportunity to see where I went: I might go nowhere, I might find it difficult to relax or sink into myself, but whatever happened, he reassured me, he could hold me.

Those words 'I can hold you' have become so deeply connected to my understanding of the Warrior, to trust and a sense of protection.

A combination of deep relaxation along with appropriate and guiding music led me into an experience I find hard to describe, but it has stayed with me and I know it will never leave me.

I went into the session with a completely open mind and heart, prepared to just feel comfortable and rested, as I might do at the end of a yoga session when I am lying on my mat, silently praying the person next to me won't fart.

First, Ryan asked if I was comfortable with touch and explained that during the session he might sense that I needed to feel reconnected to another human being just to act as reassurance or to bring me back into the room.

The breathing was nasal, entirely, apart from one gasp and frantic exhale that I am aware of in the middle, and deepest, part of the session. As my breath lengthened under Ryan's guidance, I became acutely aware of every inch of my body and where the inward breath was going.

I found that as I inhaled, I drew my breath right up from my belly, into my diaphragm, chest, throat, head and arched my neck as if I wanted it right up into the top of my head. It was an instinctive and animalistic urge to draw every single fragment of oxygen into my soul to protect me and empower me as I dived down below layers of clutter that had been there for years.

The music in the background guided me intelligently and instinctively, or maybe I was reacting to the change in tone, lyrics and intensity. As the pitch, rhythm and bass accumulated in the room, it echoed within my body. To say that it was akin to sex is not an exaggeration, nor is it suggesting there was anything happening to me other than within my own body. It started to feel as if there was a storm brewing in my chest and guts and I knew that something wanted to get out. I was feeling a mixture of fear and anger, both of which I still cannot explain, merely recount. And then my mother's wedding ring jumped across my neck on the thin gold chain that carries it. Just a tiny but definite movement, which, later, Ryan said he had witnessed too.

The feeling of disturbance and turmoil was continuing to build within me, along with a compulsion to lash out, to fight something. I felt a gentle touch on my left hand and because my eyes had been closed from the moment the session began, I could only assume it was Ryan taking my hand. I struck out; I needed to go through whatever was happening to me on my own, but then a hot rush of emotion washed over me, my face screwed up in pain and I groaned, tears squeezing out of my tightly closed eyes.

'I can hold you,' he had said. I felt Ryan's warm hand take mine once more and this time I accepted his presence. I felt whatever was inside me jump out of my body and disappear off to the right of the room. Immediately, I relaxed and tears flowed more easily.

I took a single, raw and desperate breath through my mouth and then closed it again, somehow aware that by holding on to the regular pattern of nose breathing I would stay safe and be able to guide myself back out of wherever I had been.

Ryan must have sensed that I was done. He let go of my hand and I wriggled my numb fingers to let the blood flow again. Slowly, I became aware once more of my limbs, not just my internal world. Toes wriggled happily, legs flexed and straightened. Ryan's voice and lighter music guided me back fully into the room. It took me a good few minutes to feel aware of where I was and to want to open my eyes and let any light in. I held my hands across my eyes to filter the daylight beam by beam. Nothing had changed in the room, and yet everything had changed in me. Whereas before there had been a constant chatter and questioning, now there was a pool of stillness and strength.

The second part of the day was still to come.

The ice bath, which the thermometer measured at 2 °C, awaited me out in the garden in the afternoon sunshine. I smiled. This is what I had wanted and Ryan had delivered it.

When I climb into my own tub back at home, I have virtually no ceremony of preparation, physical or mental, so today I was keen to learn the method of straw breathing, which is something Ryan has developed from his own practice. It triggers the biochemical changes required to embrace extreme cold. And provides you with a tool to hang on to when the pain of the ice bites into your brain and you just want to leap out of the galvanised steel bathtub.

We sat for around twenty minutes on the grass working through the stages of breathing until I was ready. My immersion was slow and controlled, in spite of my excitement about embracing this intense cold. I hadn't been in water/ice this cold since the winter when I lay down in a semi-frozen mountain tarn, Bowscale Tarn, in the Lake District. I think my brief, but relevant, experience in very cold water helped me to appreciate rather than fear the ice bath, so I was able to relax and enjoy every second.

The pain on my feet was intense, but by continuing to breathe in and exhale as if through a straw, I kept my movements fluid and strong. I didn't gasp or falter as I planted both feet squarely on the tub base and started to lower myself into a lying position in the broken chunks of ice. There was a moment when my brain screamed at me to get out, but I have experienced a similar automatic protective response many times during my years of winter swimming and each time have paid attention, checked I'm okay and then overridden it.

I wanted this so badly and felt completely confident about doing it. Ryan squatted down by the tub and guided me once more into the realms of the seemingly impossible with warmth, sincerity and authority.

I was in, except for the final few inches of submersion and the most difficult: the back of the neck. Ryan placed his hand against the end of the tub and told me to lean my head back against it. He gently withdrew his hand and the ice water seeped right around my skull. This triggers the mammalian response, making the blood scoot away from the peripheries and into the core to protect it. Without this trigger, the experience of being in the ice bath is far more excruciating and the benefits are significantly reduced. I wanted to feel the full force of the ice and cold, so did exactly what Ryan suggested. And then I relaxed deeply into myself, with my eyes closed and my breath regulated. At that point I couldn't hear or sense anything of my surroundings, just what was going on inside my body and the lingering, stabbing pain of the cold, mostly in my hands and feet. I barely heard Ryan ask me to open my eyes and reconnect with him. He was smiling and I smiled back. This human gesture broke the trance, and allowed my senses to kick back in too.

What a beautiful experience, to lie buried under ice, but with the warmth of a September afternoon filtering through the leaves on the overhanging branches of the beech tree.

Three minutes passed and Ryan gave me the option of climbing out, or staying in a little longer. He gets everyone out at five minutes. I didn't really want to get out, but after another minute I felt 'cooked' and slowly climbed out of the tub.

My huge grin told the world how happy and exhilarated I was! To force the blood back into my limbs I did a few horse squats and danced around in my swimsuit on the lawn. And then we sat wrapped in blankets with our hands nursing comforting mugs of hot tea and chatted some more.

I left Ryan's workshop a different person from the one who had arrived. And I brought home with me more tools to use in my own daily practice and life. At moments of stress, indecision or sadness, I now have that pool of stillness within me.

ELAINE

Elaine's hair is down to her bum and very red. She exudes calm, strength and balance. She applies these qualities to all the sports she loves: pole dancing, paddleboarding, weightlifting, cycling, running and outdoor swimming.

'I survived the night' were the first words ever spoken into my voice recorder while I lay under my duvet in Gloria, my VW campervan. I had parked her up alongside a hedge in a public car park right next to Castle Semple Loch, south-west Scotland. Looking back, I can recall the relief I felt that cold, October morning. Daybreak was peeking down through the front window of the pop top. Elaine had always insisted that I'd be fine parking in Castle Semple Visitor Centre car park for the night – it turned out she was right. After abandoning a campsite I'd booked outside Largs because it gave me a very bad feeling, in spite of rave reviews on the Pitchup website, I had reluctantly driven out of town and up into the hills. First I lost daylight, then I lost 4G. I am not sure which made me more anxious. A solo 'wild' campervan experience was not what I had anticipated or had ever tried before. The thought of parking up in the middle of nowhere on my own terrified me.

For a brief couple of minutes I considered driving the two hours home to Cumbria and then driving back up first thing in the morning. Elaine messaged me to reassure me that she had often seen other campervans in the public car park. 'You'll be fine,' she said.

Not only was I fine, but I know it did me good.

But, however excited and proud I was to have survived the night, I had come equipped for staying a night in a campsite. I had left the Porta Potty at home. This hadn't been a problem during the cover of darkness, as you can imagine, but the body is a funny thing. If it needs to go, it needs to go, and mine is as regular as my heartbeat. But here's a thing: it is possible to deliver in a bin bag. That's all I'm saying.

Apart from that, clearly, the biggest bonus of all from being parked up right at the edge of a Scottish loch is that you get to see what happens there at sunrise, and it is a busy place. First, the birds, who had finally fallen asleep after the wheel-spinning locals had receded, started preening, chattering, nuzzling and flapping stiff wings in the cool autumnal air. No one else but me was wandering around, mug of hot tea in one hand, phone in the other. It felt like I had stepped into a world of feathers, dust, quacks, splashes, honks and squawks. The sky was beginning to change colour: tangerine, shell pink, faint purple and warm grey, all reflected on to the surface of the calm loch. I wanted to join the birds, be in the loch, feel the change in light on my skin, watch the goosebumps snuggle between erect arm-hairs. Not early enough and too public for a skinny dip, I knew I had seconds to transform from human to dipper. I returned to Gloria for everything I needed, congratulating myself once again on being brave enough to bring her here in the scary darkness of the previous night.

Sunrise dips for me are more intensely experienced if solitary and private, so I walked right down to the far end of the car park, where there were a few floating jetties – I felt an urge to jump off a jetty, but good sense reminded me that I had no idea of what I was jumping into, the depth, or the bottom of the loch. Just as I was debating my entry point and removing my changing robe, in a world of my own, a deep Scottish voice said, 'Good morning, you'll be wanting to swim, then?' It was a man dressed in Lycra shorts and top carrying a scull under one arm. After a brief exchange about the best place for me to enter the water, he set his boat down a few metres from the shore and disappeared into the ever-changing sunrise colours. And I walked down a short ramp into the blackness of the loch; content that this was a good place to be. My heart was full of excitement and warmth, confirming why I love Scotland so much.

From the moment we greeted each other in the car park, my gut feeling about Elaine was realised. Her soft Scottish accent, her gentle but sure mannerisms and the way she sorted out the logistics of the morning enabled me to relax into easy conversation as she drove me to a small reservoir up in the hills above Castle Semple Loch, with only the occasional fisherman to disturb the solitude. And it is this solitude that Elaine craves. We stood on the bank, absorbing the early morning sound of silence. I was slightly apprehensive about the swim because I hate deep water and Elaine explained that there was a steep drop-off because it is an old reservoir, but we would be able to walk in down a piece of matting and keep to the shoreline if I was nervous. As we disrobed, the cool autumnal air nipped my skin and I felt a frisson of something: excitement, apprehension, curiosity, fear. I pushed it away. Elaine walked down the matting with the confidence of familiarity and I knew it was my turn. I put the GoPro on my head so that I could film us while swimming. I wanted to talk with her in situ, in the loch, in the water. So I slid down the matting as elegantly as I could, and then I was suddenly in and swimming, no idea how deep it was, but I reached Elaine's side and took up position on her left so that I was closest to the bank. As I did this, I asked the question: 'So, what is it about the cold that you love?' We both laughed, because it did feel cold and for a brief moment I know we both thought, what the hell are we doing?!

'It's that moment, like now, and I know it sounds a strange thing to love, but when I feel a sharp pain shoot up my spine, up the back of my neck. It focuses my mind. I get a solace that I just don't get anywhere else. It's not that I don't enjoy swimming with others too, but there's something about being on your own, in a place like this, just being part of it all. I suppose that's one of the reasons I come here so early in the morning, I am guaranteed the place to myself. I can watch the world waking up and share it in a really small way. It gives me a sense of connectedness I just don't find in other parts of life. Gertrude Ederle said, "When we're in the water, we're not in this world", but I feel the opposite.[3] I am not spiritual but this is as

---

3   Gertrude Ederle was the first woman to swim the Channel and she did it, in spite of everyone telling her women couldn't swim that distance, on her first attempt on 6 August 1926.

close as I get to being spiritual; I don't have other parts of my life that give this quality of peace.

'On the summer solstice I was swimming, just here, about here and I saw a roe deer leap out of the undergrowth and into the loch about twenty feet in front of me. I thought it was going to swim to the other side, but it turned and eyeballed me. I don't know whether it was more surprised or me. But it seemed to think "meh", turned and swam back to the bank and scrambled out. But what an experience!

'And I know it so well. I love coming to the same place time after time to watch the seasons change. I've been swimming here, doing lengths of the loch, straight into the sun, and just closed my eyes and gone into a kind of meditative state, lulled by the rhythm of my stroke until I reach the end. I've heard swans flying right overhead, so low; the loudness of their wings is phenomenal as I watch them pedalling across the surface of the loch coming in to land. It's made me almost want to cry with happiness.'

There is a sharpness on an autumnal morning, like that day, when the surface of the loch was glassy. My eyes were closed and I was listening to Elaine explain how she loves to be in the same place when the temperatures are starting to drop because it adds another level to the exhilaration and experience of being outdoors, so close to nature, actually in nature, as we were then. The idea that there is a continuity and evolution, the only thing that changes is our body states before and after being in the water: is that why so many swimmers take pre-swim and post-swim selfies?

Elaine had had to break ice to get in once, just thin ice, but all the same she found it exciting because the air had been so crisp and still, and she had felt her skin responding to it even before she got in the water.

'As I swam I breathed in the cold air and felt so lucky to be alive. I felt totally invigorated when I climbed out, as if I could do anything. It's like a giant wake-up call. But, I have to confess, I do love warm water! Maybe I'm not a true cold-water swimmer? I just love being in the water, moving through the water.'

Is this why you wear a wetsuit as the water temperature drops? Given that she can only come swimming once a week, she feels the need to make the most of being out and wants to stay in the water longer. 'I believe I still get the benefits of being outdoors all year round, whether I'm in a wetsuit or not. I still know it's cold, my body still responds and I still have to watch how long I'm in for.'

As we were getting close to the matting where earlier I had slid in so elegantly, I wondered if it was not the cold that fascinated her, but the combination of doing something that gets tougher and takes more mental strength to do, but also has greater benefits as a result?

'I need to swim in a way that I don't need to cycle or run. There is something about moving through the water, being immersed in nature as a single being, that elevates whatever mood I am in.' It seems to be her version of mindfulness. It makes her complete in a way that no other sports she has tried do: running gives her sore muscles and makes her feel tired; cycling gives her sore muscles and makes her feel hungry; if she is angry or frustrated, she will lift weights, as that is physically and mentally challenging, it's tough and enables her to vent her emotions.

She likes rhythm and maybe that is what is meditative about actually moving through the water. She goes into a trance-like state of repetitive movements, but not in the same way as when she is pole dancing. Then, although there is music and rhythm, it is physically gruelling and leaves your muscles sore and bruised. Swimming is the only thing that is calming and energising, physically and mentally, at the same time.

Swimming doesn't fix a problem for her, as it can do for other people, but gives her the headspace to go back to the problem once she's done swimming. She can't find that headspace when she's running or cycling as she's focusing on cadence, speed, traffic and terrain. She actually doesn't want to think when she's swimming; she wants to leave that all behind at her desk, in her house. The bizarre and notable difference between Elaine and myself is that whereas I have often gone to the water deliberately if I'm feeling angry or upset because I know it will bring me down, help me rationalise my emotions and come out feeling stronger and better able to deal with the situation or person who has created the anger, she has never gone to the water in that state, so she doesn't know how it would affect her, whether it would help her.

I noticed that her teeth were starting to chatter as I took photos of her with my GoPro: time to get out. We'd both forgotten that the air and water temperatures were actually quite chilly. There was an atmosphere about this tiny, disused reservoir that is both wild and cultivated at the same time, much like Elaine, with her incredibly long, red hair, strong presence and calm, reassuringly 'ordinary', sedentary, working-from-home life. This is her escape, her sanctuary, and I felt privileged to have been invited to join her there on such a beautiful autumnal morning.

I gazed across the water to the far side, where I thought I could see an old dwelling and a person sitting on the bank – my imagination, or images from the past, when there was indeed an old farm with real-life people working hard to make the land produce food and shelter? It reminded me of when I had walked up to Black Moss Pot in the Lake District and in my state of mild hypothermia had imagined I could see a fortress high up on the fellside. These northern landscapes, the Lake District, Scotland are places of beauty that reach far beyond skin deep. Wild, remote, strong and everlasting: places of Warriors.

MATTY

Matty's first competitive swimming event as an adult was in 2016, the Chillswim in Windermere. It was a massive turning point for him physically and mentally: he had agreed to be in a relay team as a bit of a joke, attracted by the idea of swimming in fancy dress. He went on to win silver medals, become a world champion of sorts and dance at parties in between each swim race dressed as a turkey. He almost felt as if he had cheated in some way, so he spent the next fifteen months working on his technique, cold-water adaption and resilience. Next time he wanted to feel as if he had actually earned the medals. Matty's two dreams are to win a gold medal, and for saunas and ladders into bodies of water to be a familiar sight in the UK.

Matty opened our conversation by describing a recent visit to Finland. He always spends some time swimming and taking a sauna by the lake. The following is typical of what usually happens: Matty pulls open the sauna door and its occupants groan. They are cross because his hypothermic body will bring down the temperature of the sauna (typically a Finnish sauna is kept at 70–80 °C). As he sits there shivering and trying to ignore the disgruntled whispers, he sips a hot drink. The locals shake their heads and dismiss him as 'that strange British man who stays in the water a long time'. They're not concerned about his safety, just that he brings the cold into the sauna with him. But, after many trips to Finland, Matty is now used to this reaction.

I asked him about the difference between the Finns' relationship with cold water and the UK's. It is Finnish culture to sauna and dip repeatedly, sometimes only dipping for seconds. It's less about endurance, but is more sociable and relaxing. It is something children start to do from a young age, and saunas and ladders into a small ice hole are commonplace. Air temperatures can be between -10 and -20 °C for long periods, so wooden structures are often built around a small hole at the bottom of a ladder, and sometimes warm air is blown in to keep it from freezing over. Does that mean we're more hardcore in the UK because we measure distance and time? Not necessarily, he responded. It's just it's not practical in such a cold climate to keep any extent of water unfrozen and therefore open for swimming.

He knows he brings with him a completely different attitude to the cold water. He dips, yes, and swims, but repeatedly and for longer periods than the locals. In between times, he goes into the sauna to stop his core temperature dropping below 32 °C. If there is a hot tub available he prefers this to a sauna for an immediate post-swim warm-up because it is more gentle, usually at 38–40 °C, so it works to rebalance the body rather than roast it!

Matty's approach to risk has in part grown from his work, where he faces violence and intimidation on a daily basis. His body is attuned to risk, which means he respects those who work within the emergency services and does all that he can to promote their messages and standards on his social media.

But his personal philosophy stems from earlier in his life, when he spent some of his time in the mountains of British Columbia, Canada. Here his relationship with the cold was forged. In 2004, in a glacial lake, where the water temperature was still only 5 or 6 °C in summertime, he had his first encounter with cold-water swimming. As he entered the water, he reminded himself that if he got in he'd have to get himself out: a rule he had always applied to hiking in the mountains. It's a rule he applies to every swim he does. However far his swim goal, he never steps into the water without an escape plan. A quick dip or a swim across the lake: how will he get out if there is an issue? It's fine to swim to the other side, but if he's tired, can he jog back? There have been a few occasions he can remember clearly where he had to rely on his tow float. He describes one time swimming quite a distance across a lake when he became dizzy and disoriented, and couldn't tell up from down or forward from back. By grabbing his tow float, he was able to hang on to it and float until his head had stopped spinning. Then, rather than continuing his planned swim using heads-down front crawl, he stuck to breaststroke to avoid a repeat of the disorientation.

At the end of our conversation I asked Matty, 'Is there a part of you that the cold reaches that nothing else can?'

His answer surprised and intrigued me. He had read the extensive research into the effects of cold water on dementia and applied it to his own brain and inner self. At work, he sees and experiences violence, physical and emotional, on a regular basis, because of the type of client he is involved with. Mental instability, alcohol, drugs and abuse are regular topics he has to discuss and deal with, along with life-saving strategies such as CPR and defibrillation. Life can be hanging by a thread and it is his job to catch it. The repercussions for his own mental health would be devastating if he didn't have a mechanism for creating a boundary between himself and that level of aggression.

'I go into the cold to forget things, genuinely.' When we go into the cold, our body shuts our systems down to the core essentials to keep us alive. The body thinks it's under attack, but when it thinks we're safe, it switches back on. Different switches in the brain, including the memory, are turned off and sometimes stay off. Matty finds it quite natural to think like this: a biological switching off and not back on. It is so black and white, in fact, that once, when he was a witness to a horrific crime, a cold night swim blotted it out of his memory. A few days later the police asked him to give a statement, but he genuinely couldn't remember what had happened. The trauma had been wiped from his memory and protected him from the horror repeating itself in his dreams and thoughts. It's not up to him to choose what to forget, though, he explained. His psyche lets go of things that are toxic for him, things that would do him harm emotionally and mentally before they could affect him physically. It is as if the cold water washes the dirt in his brain off. I wondered if this was only possible because he knew his body so well. It was as if his subconscious knew what to do to make him safe and cleanse him.

It's not even that much of a complicated process, he laughed, as the battery on his phone began to wane … so the last words I heard from him spoke of a double whammy. To him, it was clear and deeply connected to his Christian beliefs. First thing in the morning, he lays problems and worries at Jesus's feet and then walks away. Later, the cold water cleanses him of the day's tough situations and emotions: a form of baptism. He sees baptism as a sacrament, an exercise of putting old systems away and bringing your virtues to the fore.

However, in the echoing silence of our conversation and the black half screen where Matty had once been, large and definitely real, I sensed I had just been witness to someone who didn't actually need that daily baptism, because he didn't need to let go of himself. Immersion in the cold water kept his soul clean, untainted by the appalling work situations he was exposed to. He had a good system of personal protection: his faith, his regular cold-water exposure and his tow float.

In a message later that evening, Matty thanked the battery for dying – it had given him time to digest our conversation and summarise why he loved the cold water: 'in the same way that we flush away the body's waste products, the cold helps me wash away the brain's waste products that sleep can't seem to shift. And yes, my faith helps deal with the spiritual waste.'

JAIMIE

My final Warrior is another woman. Internationally celebrated for her incredible cold-water swimming achievements, popular public speaker and advocate for women in sport Jaimie Monahan knows the cold with every fibre of her body. However, she came to it gradually, from a background of competitive pool swimming into marathon swims that were often in cold water. The sociable, community-focused ice-swimming championships and events were as much part of the buzz as the cold itself. Solo ice swimming challenges, such as the Oceans Seven and the even more extreme Ice Sevens, became addictive to her.[4]

The image of childhood she remembers most strongly is having a red nose and ears, being wrapped up in the house and sipping hot chocolate made by her mum. There had been a big gathering in her local town to celebrate the cold season. During the winter, school would open its doors once a day so all the children could run out to roll in the snow. Good memories. Only good memories associated with the cold.

On her own, in a vast ocean, she leaves behind her celebrated name, her role as a motivator, or as a competitor. Swimming next to huge waves and towering icebergs, she is just herself, enjoying what her body can do. It becomes a mental and physical state of being where nothing else matters

4   The Oceans Seven is an extreme challenge to swim the seven long-distance open-water swims across the most dangerous sea channels in the world: Catalina Channel, USA, 21 miles; Molokai Channel, Hawaii, 28 miles; Cook Strait, New Zealand, 16 miles; Strait of Gibraltar, Spain and Morocco, 8 miles; Tsugaru Strait, Japan, 12 miles; North Channel, Great Britain and Ireland, 21 miles; English Channel, Great Britain and France, 22 miles.

    The Ice Sevens is where the swimmer has to swim a mile in each of the seven continents' oceans, all of them 5 °C or lower. One of the ice miles, Ice Zero, has to be in water below 1 °C.

except small changes setting off tiny alarm bells connected to her strength and stamina. Her only thought is to reach the end of the swim safely and to be able to walk out by herself, not in such a state of hypothermia that she needs to be carried out.

This intrigued me. It must be tempting to push yourself to the absolute limit on every challenge and rely on your support team to carry you out if necessary. But this attitude is completely the opposite of Jaimie's philosophy. Her challenges are often in remote areas geographically, where the locals may never have seen someone swimming in the ocean, let alone in the ice. It goes against her nature to cause chaos or upset. 'I swim in gently and walk out gently,' she says. 'It's my wish for everyone who undertakes such privileged challenges to respect nature, other people and themselves.'

She believes she has a responsibility to explain why cold-water and ice swimming can be dangerous, but doesn't want to stop people's joy. 'When I go into the water, I want to get out of that water, so I always check in on myself the morning of a swim: how do I feel today? Am I tired? Did I have one wine too many? Do I have the right focus?'

She has seen too many people being carried out of the water screaming in pain, putting other people's lives at risk to rescue them – and then posting about it on social media. 'Someone seeing your post might think it's normal to push yourself to the limit and see it as almost heroic, which is more worrying. It's not a competition to see how close to death you can push yourself! You get the same rush if you're in for two minutes or twenty.'

Going to a cryotherapy salon once a week for 'a nice cold shot' has made Jaimie question what her motives are for swimming in cold water: is it being immersed in stunning landscape, or icebergs, animal and bird life? Or is it the physical activity of swimming? Or spending time with friends? Or is it here in this dry, cold chamber where the pure thrill and shock of physical sensations are artificially created, but no less real and beneficial? Before using cryotherapy she wouldn't have been able to separate the physical from the mental or emotional, but in the chamber she can experience the pure cold. You're given woolly boots, gloves and hat to protect your peripheries from frostbite because the chamber gets to -140 °C. You're only allowed to stay in for three minutes, which is enough.

You also wear a surgical mask to make sure you're not breathing in unfiltered cold, but she loves to take one deep breath to really feel it. If you didn't know what to expect, it could be shocking. Your body reacts the same way: that sharp intake of breath, the settling and relaxing, the shivering and the same giddiness afterwards.

Sitting still for three minutes in the cryo chamber is not something she'd be able to do if she was in water. The only time she is forced to be still is holding on to the ladder just before the start of a race, and for her this is the hardest part because she doesn't know what to do with her body if it is not moving, how to deal with the cold and the almost immediate shivering. As soon as the gun goes, she moves and transitions from her mind into her body, which knows exactly what to do and how to overcome the challenges of the race: the distance, the location, the solitude, whatever situation she is in. It's a 'moving meditation' and is her most natural state of being. I imagine her as a selkie, shedding all human awkwardness and becoming streamline, at one with the water and aquatic life around her.

And once there, alone in the cold water, she appreciates how small she feels in the big scheme of things. It is an intriguing dichotomy which draws her back to remote locations in search of something deeper than the physical sensation of being cold. There, swimming next to a massive iceberg, she feels in touch with something primal, whereas in urban Manhattan, her home, she is never further than a metre or so from another human being. If we never feel this solitude, how can we understand our place in nature, our vulnerability, and nature's too? Humans have had an immense impact on the planet; ecosystems and balance have been disturbed. As Jaimie said, we can't ever hope to understand how deep this impact goes unless we experience our smallness and insignificance. One way to do this is to spend time alone in nature. Here, a deep sense of humility and gratitude will work their way into our souls.

I thought I'd understood how I see my Warrior, but Jaimie took it to another level. She taught me that to be a true Warrior you need a daily reference to the real world. Ice swimmers often talk about fighting the cold, defeating the cold, as if they are working against the challenge rather than with it. When she's out in the Southern Ocean battling her way through choppy water, scraping her arm against an iceberg, freezing her face and squinting through tiny goggles at a dark shape in front of her, fears of killer whales and hungry bull seals threatening to sink her, it won't help to fight because she's just too small in this huge scale of nature. Instead, she has to find the mental strength to calm her breath, get out of her head and back into her body, trust her experience and the experience of the team supporting her.

I told her about the day my mum died and how I had gone to my place of ghosts and ended up walking right round Crummock Water, further than I had walked for years. I had pictured a Warrior walking next to me, shadowing me, there to encourage me when I hesitated or wanted to give up.

'That was you, your Warrior. Everyone can be their own Warrior,' said Jaimie.

THE
CHILD

My Child is a shy individual, who has a strong sense of
curiosity about the world and other people, but doesn't always
have enough self-confidence to match her dreams. She watches
from the sidelines, longing to join in the games, but not quite
daring to. Occasionally, she bursts out of this shell and
persuades other people to do what she wants to do.
Her enthusiasm for life and fun is infectious and it is as
if in those moments she is able to forget her shyness.

A gentle and caring individual, whose smile lights up a room,
but who often looks away or down at the ground. She is content
to play on her own, using her imagination to create worlds and
scenarios, but longs to have more friends to play with.

There is something intrinsically open, honest and innocent about
her view of the world and how she wants to be in the world. Full
of energy and constantly fidgeting and moving around, but with
no need to raise her voice to attract attention. Natural to look at,
natural in her behaviour and connection to the world around her.

RORY

Rory is built for running up fells, not swimming in cold lakes; he has an amazing power-to-weight ratio, which has enabled him to run up most of the mountains and fells in the Lake District, but no spare flesh around his bones to protect him from the low water temperatures he has endured on many of his recent challenges, such as the Deep Tarn Project in 2020.[5] Originally from a running background, with a plethora of personal challenges ticked off, Rory is constantly active and planning his next adventure, project or challenge. His energy is evident as soon as you meet him and his natural curiosity for facts, figures and statistics drives him to try new sports, support different causes and collaborate in a variety of business and personal ventures.

Rory has suffered from a couple of difficult injuries, which have led him into open-water swimming because it is a low-impact but high-focus activity that suits his nature and recovery needs. In 2018, I was lucky enough to be one of a handful of Lake District swimmers who became involved at the start of his water journey. I'll never forget his face as he lowered himself into Whisky Pool for the first time! It was definitely a baptism by chilli prickles. Fortunately, it didn't put him off his goal, which was to educate himself from within the outdoor swimming community about safety, gear, swim location, biosecurity and swim etiquette. We all wanted to facilitate amazing experiences for him because we could see his determination and ability. But what has always astonished me about Rory is his dedication to

---

5   The Deep Tarn Project was completed in 2020 (but started in 2019), and involved swimming the length of all twenty of the Lake District tarns deeper than ten metres during the winter swim season.

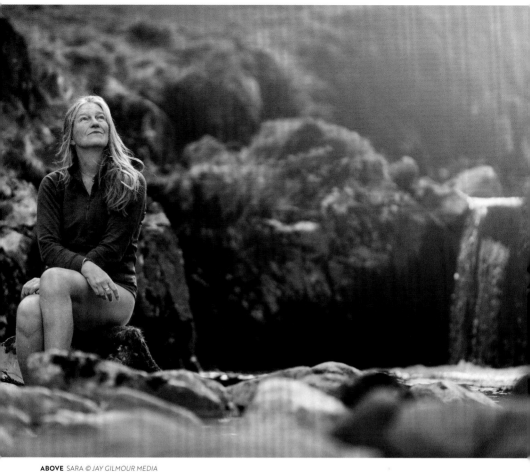

ABOVE SARA © JAY GILMOUR MEDIA

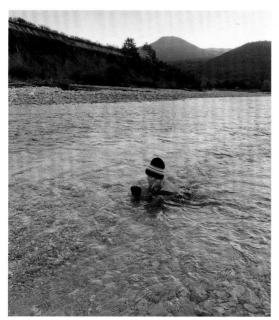

ABOVE CLAUDIA © SARA BARNES

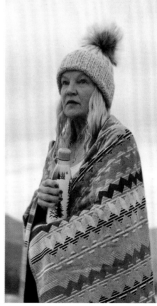

ABOVE CLAUDIA © CLAUDIA

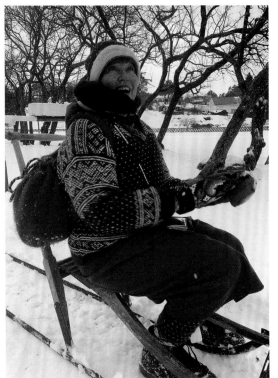

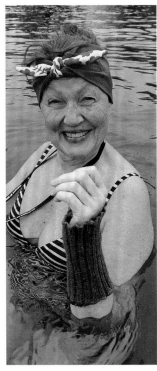

LEFT & ABOVE SOLVEIG © SARA BARNES

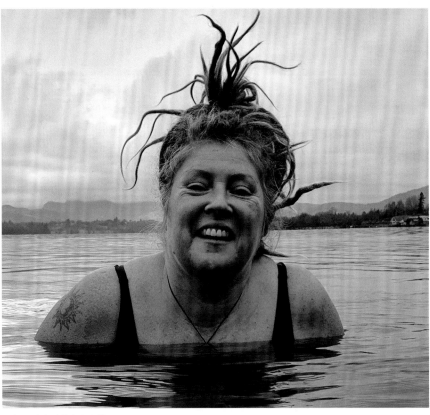

ABOVE LEELOU © SARA BARNES

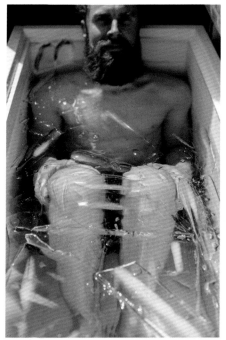

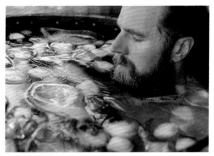

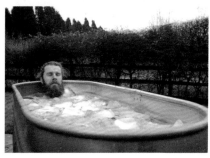

LEFT & TOP RIGHT RYAN © *EMMA LEDWITH*
ABOVE RYAN © *JACK TEW*

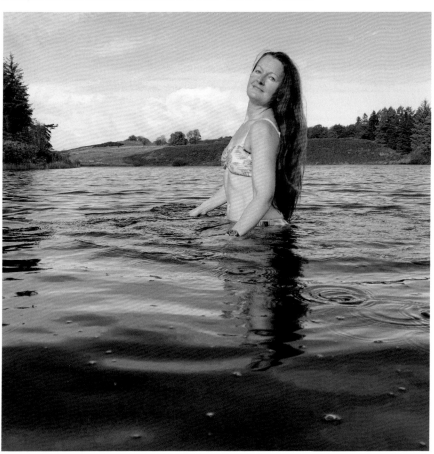

ABOVE ELAINE © *SARA BARNES*

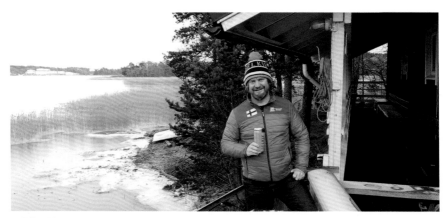

ABOVE *MATTY © TANJA-MARIA LAAKSO*

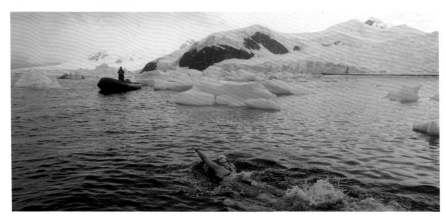

ABOVE & BELOW *JAIMIE © ARIK THORMAHLEN*

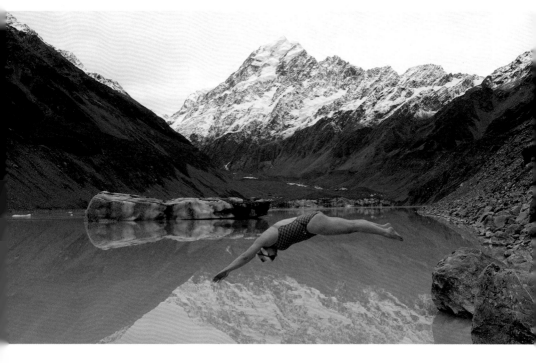

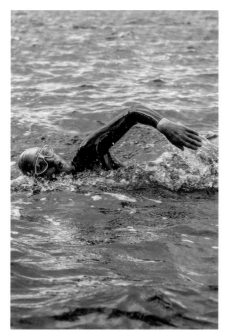

ABOVE RORY © GARTH DEW

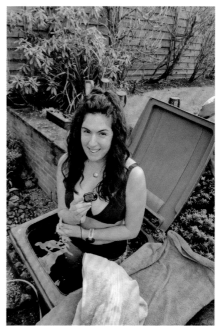

ABOVE SARAH © SARAH GROVES

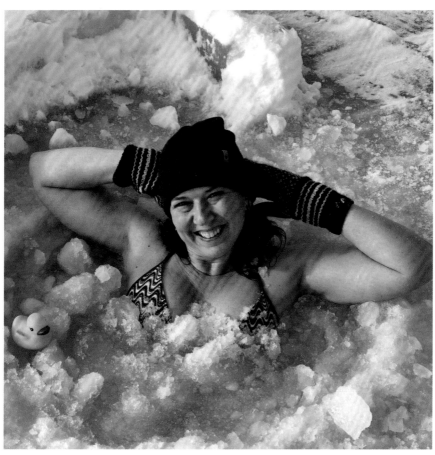

ABOVE ELLI © BETTI BERNTSEN

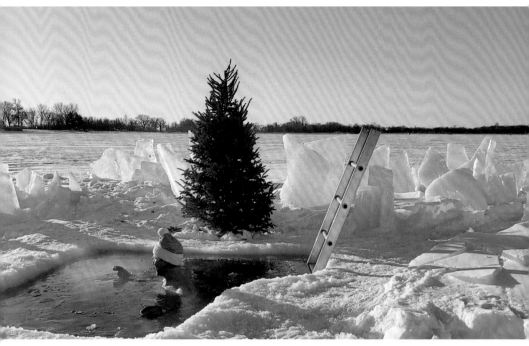

ABOVE JOHNNIE © *JOHNNIE SCHMIDT*

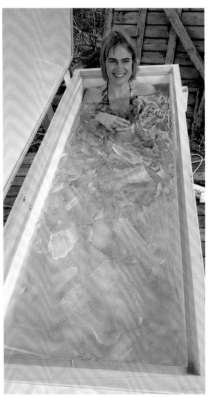

ABOVE FIEN © *FIENTJE LEERMAN*

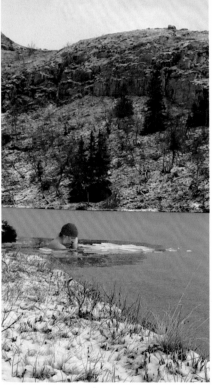

ABOVE JAY © *JASON BRYAN*

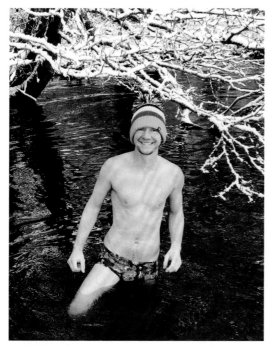

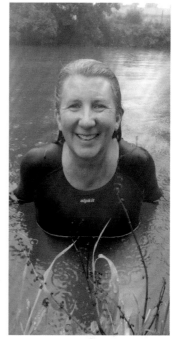

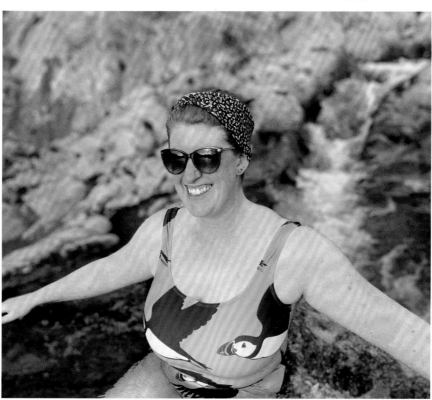

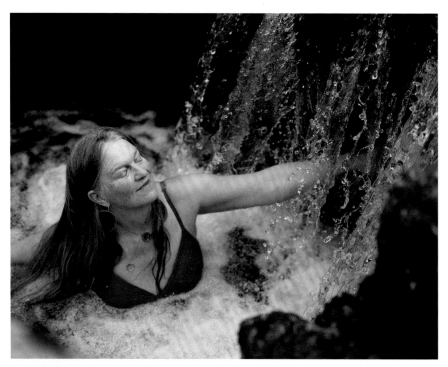

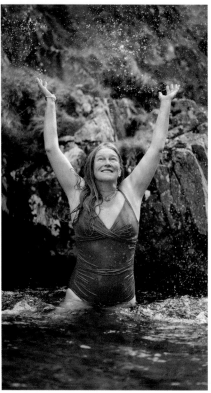

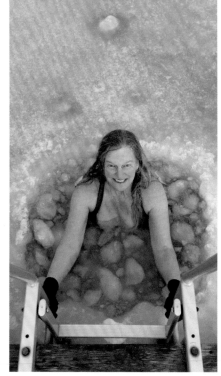

TOP & ABOVE SARA © *JAY GILMOUR MEDIA*   **ABOVE** SARA © *JASON BRYAN*

whatever project he undertakes, both in terms of personal safety and his thorough research and recording of the facts. His 'process' is critical to him and if he deviates from it, he almost immediately feels insecure and uncomfortable.

Back to where it all started: Crummock Water in the North-West Lakes on a blustery end-of-January day. Steely grey water that looked about as inviting as … actually, it's just the sort of weather to go swimming, if you enjoy being bounced about in slappy waves, buffeted by the spindrifts that whistle down the lake and chilled to the bone by the brutal wind as you walk back out to the bench by the woods.

I really don't care what anyone else wears to swim in so long as we are all comfortable in what we are wearing. Skins (as in just a swimsuit) or wetsuit – we are both going to feel the cold and get cold, one of us more quickly than the other, but most importantly we are both standing here on a winter's day laughing and chatting as we complete our preparations to walk into the lake. High five and we're off. The moment of cold water against flesh isn't synchronised, but I can see that Rory is as focused on entering the water as I am; we both need to mentally adjust from being warm and dry to being cold and wet. Our methods are different: Rory splashes water on the back of his neck, pulls down his goggles, sights right down the far end of the lake and then swoops in head first and starts to swim. I, on the other hand, wince a bit, hug myself or hold my elbows out of the water and then talk myself round to spreading my arms out so my hands are just skimming the surface of the water. That way, my body is completely exposed to the water and I take the hit all at once as I submerge and then push off with my feet and I'm in. Rory has stopped and turned round to swim back to meet me. Then, together, we try to swim through bouncy waves, unable to chat because if we did we'd swallow half the lake. It is fun and bracing. I know I won't be in as long as Rory, but I've never had a problem with getting out when I'm ready. I don't feel pressure to stay in for as long as other people.

Reaching the shallow water, Rory keeps his word and takes off his wetsuit. He's going to swim skins with me. It's something he has been building up gradually as he has drawn to the end of his Penguin Ninja

Challenge, toying with the idea of revisiting the Deep Tarns Project, but this time doing it in skins and maybe in the summer months.[6]

But, unlike most winter swimmers, Rory doesn't love the cold or feeling cold. For him, swimming in the cold months is about solitude and peace. The cold drives other people away, so he can experience the water and mountains on his own. Swimming heads-down front crawl, occasionally breaststroke, in the dark, blocks out everything so that he can focus on movement through the water. Years of solo night running and cycling have given him great night vision and a respect for and understanding of navigating in the dark on high mountain routes.

The challenge for him is getting up to the tarn and back down again safely, not just the cold, dark, solitude and clock. By dressing head to foot in neoprene, complete with neoprene swim hat, mitts and boots, he can swim the distance he wants to achieve in relative safety and comfort. He doesn't want to feel cold, he doesn't enjoy all the other sensations usually extolled by other swimmers. No brain freeze? There have been odd occasions where he's noticed a clamping round his head, but the hat really helps and so does consistency in doing heads-down front crawl: adaptation to the cold.

There is a certain amount of community pressure to swim skins all year round, but Rory has always had the mental strength to do his own thing, follow his own process and not get caught up in what others are or are not doing. However, as he came to the end of the Penguin Ninja Challenge the

6   Every winter, between the beginning of November and end of March, there is a Polar Bear Challenge and all the variations that have grown up around this concept, which is to swim a certain distance each month with no neoprene, just an ordinary silicone swim cap and swimming costume or trunks. The Penguin Challenge was designed for those who wanted to continue through the winter months, but who didn't feel experienced or confident enough to ditch the neoprene altogether. It gave people the opportunity to support their 'Polar Bear' friends, so no one felt alone or excluded. It has gone a long way to dispel the myth that you aren't a true outdoor swimmer if you wear neoprene – of course you are. Many swimmers joke, 'if you take your feet off the bottom of the river or lake, then you're swimming'.

Penguin Ninja was swimming three kilometres in total a month, plus these set swims at certain temperatures: 1) 1,500 metres at 9 °C or less; 2) 2,000 metres at 9 °C or less; 3) 1,250 metres at 8 °C or less; 4) 1,750 metres at 8 °C or less; 5) 1,000 metres at 7 °C or less; 6) 1,500 metres at 7 °C or less; 7) 750 metres at 6 °C or less; 8) 1,250 metres at 6 °C or less; 9) 450 metres at 5 °C or less; 10) 1,000 metres at 5 °C or less.

temptation to revisit the bite of the cold became too great.[7] Always on the lookout for a new challenge and the makings of a new project, he debated whether it was time to transition to skins and test out his now considerable cold-water swimming experience. So, he has made a conscious effort to get in the water and increase his tolerance each time, gradually building up distance and time. But again, he needs movement; he does not want to just sit in the cold water or an ice hole, and he admits he is highly unlikely to fall in love with the sensations of bordering on hypothermia time after time. His mind needs movement to focus; his fast metabolism and low heart rate of thirty-eight beats per minute is designed for cardio sports with speed and activity, not contemplation and Zen.

Because many of his Deep Tarn Project swims were in the dark, on his own and in winter, the landscape is relatively unimportant to him, so it was not a distraction from his mission, which was to run up to the tarn, set up his two scope lanterns as his reference points at one end of the tarn, walk round to the other end in his wetsuit with his running gear in his tow float and then swim the length of the tarn, guided by his two lights. He tends to swim out into the middle of a tarn where it is consistently deep because in the dark he can't see the rocks or shallow shelves around the edges. He has banged his head on rocks too many times and it always throws him off his swim.

Dark water, dark night and intense cold surrounded him. Many people questioned his decisions about personal safety, but Rory knew that his process worked – if he followed it, all would be well. A crucial, but seemingly tiny, reason for undertaking the swims at night was that no one else would be around to walk in front of his lights. If those lights vanished, he would be alone in the middle of a deep tarn with no clue where the shore was – that would terrify him, and it had happened on a couple of occasions, so he had taken the decision to always swim alone or with someone who respected his lights. Other aspects of his process include a specific wetsuit from Speedo which he can peel off like a skin, quickly and

---

7   The next challenge Rory will be doing is the Polar Bear Gold Challenge in winter 2022–23, so he is going to try and ditch the wetsuit. He's also hoping to race the 450-metre distance at the Scottish Winter Swim Championships in March 2023.

with no danger of ripping. Ease of dressing and undressing are paramount both before and after a swim – he's hot from running up to the tarn, so he can cool down more quickly as he changes into his wetsuit. He is then cold at the end of his swim and needs to get stripped off and back into running gear as quickly as possible. Unlike most other cold-water swimmers, Rory does not have a hot drink. In fact, he rarely consumes hot drinks – they are just not his thing. So, he only has his own rewarming ability and the movement of running to push round his blood once he exits the water.

Mitts, seven-millimetre neoprene, ensure he can still use his hands when he gets out of the water. Claw hands can't function and in the time it might take to warm them enough to be able to work a zip, pull off a wetsuit and redress, Rory's body would lose residual heat, putting him firmly in the danger zone. To always have someone else with him to help him get dressed would go against his philosophy, which is that if he gets himself up the mountain and into the water, he has to be able to get himself back out and down to his car under his own steam without unnecessary drama or risk to himself or anyone else. It's all part of the challenge and commitment to himself and his project. It brings a focus that nothing else does: the cold, the dark and the solitary experience. If he can't use his hands to get dressed, he could die. He is totally self-reliant.

For him, the benefits of cold-water swimming have also been about reduction of pain from old injuries, particularly when he first started and had a reoccurring foot injury, which was preventing him from his regular running routines.

Everything is recorded precisely, even the short swim we had in Crummock Water. It was a statistic which will form part of his process, allowing him to continue on his journey to who knows where on the spectrum of cold-water swimming. If it's not the cold per se that intrigues him and draws him back again and again, then it is surely the magical combination of mental and physical strength working in sync against the harshest of environments, on his own, with one ultimate goal: to make a game out of the maths, a game that reverberates around his conscious as he strokes through deep, dark, cold water high above sleeping villages, watched only by creatures that inhabit lonely Lakeland tarns and fells.

They see his tall, lean figure approaching up the footpath and welcome his calm but uncomplicated presence into their realm. He leaves no trace, disturbs no one and nothing, light-footed and light-hearted, expecting nothing because he has it all within himself.

SARAH

Sarah is proof that you can get the cold fix even if you don't have a frozen lake within walking or driving distance. Although she's an experienced cold-water swimmer and normally swims in the River Avon near her home in the Midlands, circumstances in 2020 forced her to seek an alternative way of getting her daily cold immersion. A simple garden wheelie bin filled from the outside tap and topped up with ice from the freezer compartment became not just a fun thing to try, but an unexpected way of connecting with friends, family and the cold-water swimming community.

'How did I fall in love with a large, green, plastic wheelie bin?' Sarah blushes now, but from January 2021, in the third national lockdown, she began a new relationship with cold water. It was an intense, passionate affair that lasted only a couple of months, but left its mark on Sarah forever. Every morning she woke thinking about this new lover. Suddenly, she had a purpose, whereas previously every day had merged into another beige day of working from home with no physical connection to her work colleagues, family or friends. Her husband was very understanding of her new companion and together they made sure she would be safe on the patio and had everything she needed within easy reach.

Her memories of this two-month affair with her garden wheelie bin are bittersweet: her first time winter dipping was in a wheelie bin, not in a lake or river; the first time she broke ice was when the water in the bin froze over and she got a rock and smashed through; her first snowy dip was sitting submerged up to her ears in her wheelie bin, catching snowflakes on her tongue like a child. Like most other people during this third, and potentially more ominous, national lockdown, Sarah was fearful about how long it would last, and whether there was any point in getting out of bed at all to face yet another day of confinement and disconnection.

She had seen other people cleaning out wheelie bins and filling them with water during the first lockdown, almost as a kind of joke and escape from reality, but had not been interested in doing the same. But, as December slipped into a bleak January, she knew her mental health was suffering: no energy, a lack of focus, a loss of sense of humour and negative thought processes replacing her usual playful and optimistic nature.

From the moment she first climbed into her bin, she began to heal. Each morning she set her intentions for the day, starting with a dip in the bin where she gave herself permission to switch off from all thought and just enjoy physical sensations as the cold water touched every part of her body. It became a habit to video her dips, and watching them afterwards she noticed everything about her facial expressions, how her body moved and reacted to the cold water. It was as if she was testing her body on a daily basis to see what her tolerance was, what her limits were. She deliberately lowered herself slowly and focused on how it felt, until she got to her shoulders. Such a difficult part of her body to get under the water, but she did it and it got marginally easier each time.

Sarah believes that as a woman your body can experience different sensations each day because your hormones are in constant flux. The daily cold bath allowed her to get to know the moods of her body, its state of health and responsiveness, its strengths and weaknesses and its sensitivity or stoicism. So, although her brain was like a blank slate each morning, by committing to a clear and simple regime of swimsuit, hot chocolate, camera set-up, bin, breathing, it was not a dormant blank slate: it was fertile and ready to focus.

'I've always been a lover of warmer climates and I enjoy being warm. I can sit in a hot bath for over an hour! It is so bizarre that I voluntarily sat in a wheelie bin filled with cold water every day and enjoyed it!' With the world living digitally for months on end, Sarah made a point of introducing her bin to her friends and family so they could share her experience vicariously. She had no idea how involved distant relations would become or how much interest everyone would take in what she was doing. But the connections were forged and reforged every time she sat in the bin in the rain, feeling joyful in spite of the weather and sharing that spirit with others.

As the lockdown ended and the promise of better weather had her dreaming of returning to the river and even exploring further afield, she and the bin went through 'a conscious uncoupling' (to quote Gwyneth Paltrow). They went their separate ways, knowing they would come back to each other at some point in the future.

I wonder if she really would ever meet up with her bin again, or has she found a replacement? 'Nothing could replace it,' she says. 'I am still bewildered by how I managed to stick with it every day for nearly two months. I expected nothing from it, but it gave me so much. It was far more than I ever intended it to be. One of the things I noticed was how much time I spent looking at my body on the video afterwards. Not in a vain way, just curious to actually see what I look like. Maybe it's a bit like exposure therapy? Seeing myself in a swimsuit every day, not posing, just climbing inelegantly in and out of a wheelie bin. No one can look sexy doing that now, can they?! But I did! Sometimes I thought to myself, "you've got nice legs" or "good cleavage" – things I've never ever believed about myself.'

Body confidence in men and women takes such a battering because of all the unrealistic images we see every day on social media and in real life. What if we turned that on its head and asked ourselves the question: what can my body do? This is what Sarah found herself admiring. She realised that from her teens she had been so hard on herself, unforgiving even. Those lumps and bumps she hated became more tolerable every time she reran the video, or froze a frame. It was almost as if her body was shouting at her to give it a break. How could she criticise its wobbly bits and then expect it to go from warm bed to freezing bin?

As the day of release approached, Sarah's excitement to be back in the river quadrupled – snow was forecast and this added to the anticipation. Photographs of a place called The Swamp (real name Swan Pool), looking like a picture postcard in deep snow, imprinted on her brain. She had to go there! She needed to be back in nature, not a plastic bin. On the river bank the next day, scouting for a safe entry point, she heard a man call out to her, 'You're not going in, are you?' For answer, she spun round slowly, opened out her Dryrobe and revealed her swimsuit-clad body. It was more than her heckler could take. The man yanked on his dog's lead and walked away as quickly as he could.

The river was only 2 °C and burnt her body as she submerged into its flow: geese flying low across the field, sunlight picking out the snow crystals balanced on skeletal branches along the river bank, the oiliness of the cold water as her gloved hands pulled through its greenness. She remembers half closing her eyes and just becoming the water; feeling a mix of emotions rising up inside her and then wafting away into the air. A sense of being unrooted, free to move and flow exactly where she wanted, wherever the connection between the physical and the emotional took her. 'Water can be fierce and dangerous, or gentle and subdued. You're never in the same bit of water twice; it's always moving and you can't capture it.' Even in the wheelie bin she describes how at one she felt with the water itself: she could never touch the water twice in the same place; if it overflowed as she climbed in, there were bits of it she would never know or feel, a bit like life. Even if she kept completely still in the bin, the water would still move around her body as she breathed or a nerve made her twitch.

Her relationship with water has always been strong and she has always swum. But when she is actually moving through cold water, it is an exercise of distance and time for her, rather than noticing and appreciating the cold. The temperature is almost irrelevant because her focus is on where she wants to swim to and how fast she wants to get there. It is only when she is sitting still in cold water that she feels a flood of emotions being brought to the surface: everything that is crammed into her heart and mind, allowing her to release negative thoughts. As water is always in flux, she has never felt rooted to one place and has moved many times, not afraid of change and needing variety to remain stimulated. She sees life like a river: constantly flowing and if you are in it, you become part of its journey with different phases and moments, speeds and eddies, twists and bends, sometimes with debris blocking your way trying to stop you moving downstream.

The cold intensifies everything, but also clears her mind of all thought, allowing free flow of emotion to rise and fall. She has never felt more present than when sitting in her wheelie bin or in an eddy in the river.

'It's like putting the pause button on to give yourself a break, then when you get out and start to warm up, thoughts start to flow again. You don't even have to press the start button. It happens automatically. You are reset by something else beyond your control.'

THE PANTHER

Our physical and sexual self: strong, bold, playful and fierce.
Aware of all the senses and uses them to the full. Highly
motivated by physical activity and physical pleasure, but also
content to stretch lazily in the sun, enjoying admiration from
others and appreciating beauty in nature and others.
Connected to body confidence and not shy
to use physicality to express oneself.

ELLI

Elli is a collector of moments. She lives in southern Norway and tries to dip daily from a small rocky pier that juts out into the end of a fjord. I travelled to Norway in the hope of hanging off her ladder against the backdrop of a stunning sunrise.

As the Norwegian plane descended through the darkening clouds, I strained to look out of the window, not really liking what I saw: miles and miles of frozen landscape, monochrome and unwelcoming, a bit like my thoughts. I just wanted to stay on the plane in the warm, with people to look after me. As soon as I got off the plane, the uncertainty of my journey would start. No one would be there to meet me in this foreign country as I walked into the arrivals hall and stood by the carousel to wait for my two suitcases. Taxi it was. But a snowstorm was creating chaos across Norway, with flights to the north cancelled and taxis not running as frequently as normal. I'd booked a hotel in a small coastal town about fifty minutes' drive away, but it was where I had arranged to meet Elli the next day, so it seemed logical to get there that night and be able to sleep soundly knowing I'd done all the awkward transitioning and could relax.

If it hadn't been for a kind Norwegian businessman who was also waiting for a taxi, I am not sure what would have happened that Friday night at Kristiansand Airport. The benches didn't look that comfortable, but I'd have given them a shot rather than standing out in the snow waiting for the magic disappearing taxi! But the man looked after me by speaking to the taxi firm and waiting until the taxi actually arrived, forty minutes later. I felt like crying with relief as I settled into the front seat next to a fairly friendly taxi driver who clearly knew how to drive at speed on snow!

This sort of weather would bring many countries to a grinding, messy halt, but although it was causing a few travel issues, four-wheel drive and studded tyres do make a difference. How else would you go round a roundabout at forty miles per hour without spinning off into oblivion? I was tempted just to shut my eyes and cross my fingers, but in a perverse way I was soaking up the adventure and wanting him to drive faster!

The snow in Lillesand was so thick you could barely make out parked cars and there was no difference between the sky and the ground – everything was white or twinkly with thousands of fairy lights strewn across white wooden houses. If I hadn't been so desperately tired and emotional I might have found it beautiful. I cursed all the clothes I'd brought with me as I lugged two suitcases up two flights of stairs to my room. The first thing I did was peek out of the window: nothing much to see, but I could hear the gentle sound of snow still falling on snow and faint music coming from the harbour area. After a pee of relief and washing my hands, I reached for one of my duty-free bottles of wine – this called for some serious celebration. I had arrived under my own steam; I could do this. I was starving and ripped open the packets of Greek flatbreads, mature cheddar slices and Italian salami, Sainsbury's finest.

With my sense of humour slowly returning, I thought about why I was there, and when that led down some paths that seemed a bit uncertain, I told myself to stop thinking and just do. Do what? Go for a wander down to the water with my swimsuit and begin my Norwegian adventure the right way, immersing in cold water.

I had brought my fairy lights, but not the jar I usually curl them up in to create my jar of lights, which represent all the people I care about, but can't be with. A white cotton beanie is more travelproof and allows their gentle glow to be seen from a distance and give me a hug. I thought about walking into the dark water on a tiny beach, but fear gripped me: I didn't know this place, I had no idea what I was walking into and I just couldn't do it. Instead, I set my hat of lights down at the water's edge and took a photograph.

Norwegian breakfast isn't relatable to the breakfast I had imagined; in fact, some of it was unidentifiable and I had to take a tiny nibble to check what it was. Mostly cold scrambled egg, very crisp purple bacon, wilted lettuce, cucumber and red pepper. I layered this with sliced cheese on top of crunchy crispbreads and washed it down with lukewarm black coffee and orange juice. But it filled my belly and calmed my nerves a little about meeting Elli, my first host, who was picking me up from the hotel shortly.

And then everything became so much easier. I was no longer on my own wondering what the hell I was doing, but part of a family home which was warm and inviting, and immediately put me at ease and made me smile for the first time for days, it seemed.

Wrapped in this layer of warmth, I felt protected from the other, less reassuring emotions I carried with me. We swam with a small group that afternoon back in Lillesand, and drank hot chocolate afterwards standing around a few logs burning on the snowy beach. I felt I was in a different world; we just don't do it like this back home – fires are prohibited, feared by authority, not a thing of joy.

Open hearts and minds lazed around on squidgy sofas until evening and the promise of a night swim from Elli's pier before supper. The wind had picked up and sleet streaked across the windows, but this sort of weather doesn't stop swimming; it enhances the experience! And makes men out of mice, except this mouse nearly turned into a drowned rat. We walked down between the trees, across the icy road and through some more trees to a rocky drop, where Elli gave me her hand for balance. There was no easy way down to the shore and that's when the nightmare began. Imagine balancing across a series of rocks with water in between them to reach a narrow wooden walkway attached by ropes to a floating wooden jetty that juts out into the end of a fjord. Now add pitch-black night skies, a wind strong enough to straighten curly hair and ice on everything you dare to balance on. I was petrified and held Elli's outstretched hand until we were both standing on the far end of the jetty, by a lobster pot. I saw the stainless steel ladder I had so envied and desired to hold, but felt nothing but panic. Time to remove our swim cloaks and boots – we had everything else we needed; our skin was waterproof. I've not often been naked in front of people other than a partner, but I'm not body shy; to me it feels perfectly natural and far more practical to bathe naked. But with the cold wind blasting my nipples until I thought they might fall off and threatening to turn my eyes inside out, a layer of Lycra might have felt a tiny bit protective. All I had on were neoprene swim socks, gloves and a woollen hat. Elli set up her phone on a tripod and I don't know whether I was more worried about it blowing away or terrified of lowering myself down the swaying rungs of the ladder into the dark, chaotic water below.

I remember screaming and swearing a lot, from panic, exhilaration and sheer pleasure: call me perverted but this really spoke to something deep within my soul and I wanted to shout out at all the people who have hurt me over the years, 'You fuckers! Look at me now!' My gloved hands gripped the ladder tight, but eventually I let go and tried to swim towards Elli, both of us buffeted by waves and wind. We were yelling at each other and shrieking – at that moment a wonderful bond was created. She had drawn me into her world and was bobbing beside me now, at that moment more Child than Panther, but with Warrior-like compassion and strength: characteristics all intertwined into one beautiful human being.

And the wine slipped down so easily on our return to the house, our cheeks on fire and our bellies stoked with hearty casserole. The conversations continued into the night between the three of us: Elli, her partner, Kristian, and me. Years separated us, but common experiences in love and life united us – the water had brought us together, but actually now was just letting our natures and characters flow.

Elli bathes every morning, often at sunrise, from 'the walk of death'. The routine is important to her because it gives her body and mind a clean slate and opens the possibilities for the rest of the day. On windy and wet days it isn't easy to leave the house, but she has never regretted going in; she always comes out feeling refreshed and happy.

'I am a collector of moments. I make sure I am present in the moment, in the cold. My philosophy is to try to live for today because your world could fall apart tomorrow. I have had a lot of experience with grief, which is relevant to why I want to live in the moment. If you have a lot of struggles and challenges in your life that you can't necessarily do anything about, I strongly believe that this shouldn't stop you from being happy. If I have big worries, I try to allow them to be big worries and be present in that moment and then let them go. I collect the happy moments to shore up the bad times.'

One winter Elli felt crushed and wanted to just lie in the foetal position under her duvet all day; her body was begging her to leave it be, let it stay in protect mode, but she had already started cold-water swimming with the lodger in her Airbnb, so she just committed to do it every day as a way of trying to accomplish one thing at least each day, to bank the moment.

Even though she is often only in the water for three minutes, it is a twenty-minute daily experience: the anticipation, the being in, the getting out, feeling the adrenaline rush, coffee, fire, so much more than those three minutes. So, even though at that time Elli felt like she wanted to die, she was so happy in that moment: it was very pure, almost like attending a chapel of you. You are the chapel and you are paying homage to yourself. Giving yourself that time. She feels it puts everything on a different dimension to shitty life. She describes how on the one-year anniversary of her first dip, she was on a business trip, alone, swimming in a new place. It was dark and scary, but after her swim she went and got sushi as a way of trying to boost herself and celebrate. As she was eating the sushi, a thought occurred to her: just as she eats ginger to clear her palate before sushi, her cold baths are the ginger in her life: cleaning her palate ready for the day.

And if she couldn't get that cold fix? Elli explained how in the summer she fills two old bathtubs in the garden with ice once a week, but although it's cold, she doesn't experience that same fast, sharp cold she can only get from being fully immersed from her ladder. She craves the cold water, craves the endorphins and the reset she gets in the winter. Yes, it's lovely to be able to go for a swim every morning during the warmer months and she has experienced some beautiful sunrises, but the water is at least 20 °C, so she doesn't get any of the 'oooh, it's coming up my back now' feeling. There is a relaxed, fresh feeling, but not the chemical reaction that gives your body the need to do something to warm itself up. For her, it just leaves her feeling as if she's had some therapeutic exercise, but she wants to go deeper into herself, which is only possible when the temperature drops.

I've heard other swimmers talk excitedly about looking forward to the water getting colder; each day they measure the temperature and report back in anticipation: 12°, ooh getting colder; 11° today, yay! But surely there's a cut-off point to how long you can stay in the water at any temperature. Can't you just stay in the water for longer when it's warmer and get the same benefit? I know the answer to this, of course, but I'm curious to explore how a certain temperature can be a stimulant and a relaxant at the same time, and is this magic temperature different for everyone? I've noticed that at 7 °C I start to feel the difference, and from then until 5° each degree colder is a degree closer to flipping the switch.

For Elli, having studied the videos she takes on each dip, the difference is obvious: below 5° her whole face changes. It is a free facelift. If she has a migraine, the effect of the cold water can be even more dramatic: tense and pale, eyes closed and then, as she sinks down into the water and breathes slowly, her face relaxes and lifts simultaneously and she is able to open her eyes. Somehow the cold brings a change of state and emotion, which is enough to calm the migraine and give her moments of respite.

When we swam the next morning with her partner, all of us nude, I asked them both how they felt about their bodies and how nudity is seen differently in different cultures. For Elli, it's complex: she believes that we don't need fancy gear to start outdoor swimming, 'We have everything we need, we were born ready to swim,' she said, pointing at her bare skin. But society views nudity as sexual in most countries and cultures, so we hide ourselves and develop awkwardness around being naked with other people, even our sexual partners sometimes. No wonder body confidence issues are so entrenched in many societies now. Elli uses her bathing videos to alter her own perception of her body, which for years she hated and despised, not because of how it looked, but because of how she blames it for having let her down on one desperate occasion. In our conversations, she had shared some of the details of this heartbreaking story of a lost life with me, so I understood immediately the significance of the beautiful, but haunting, clay figure which she gently took down from a shelf and carried over to me. It was a woman, Elli, curled over as if trying to disappear into herself. Her still-rounded stomach was rippled and her arms were wrapped around her chest and reached round her back, the fingers nearly touching – the strength, the tragedy and the sorrow tangible.

And I thought of how she is now, hanging by one hand and foot from her ladder, stretching proudly out above the dark, cold water, naked, strong and bold. Did her daily baths do this for her? Help her unfold and reveal herself to the world? Empower her after personal loss; turn grief into moments to add to her collection?

I held that perfect clay embodiment of human emptiness as if it was my own grief, my own disappointments, my own wish for fulfilment and happiness. I have the key too; I know how the cold takes me deep within myself and scrubs out the sadness, replacing it with good, with willpower and fearlessness.

JOHNNIE

Johnnie practises cold-water immersion all year round: a chest freezer in the summer months and the ice hole he maintains in his local lake during the winter months. Creative, musical and well travelled, he feels deeply rooted to this borderland place in Minnesota: hot in summer, desperately cold and windswept in winter.

'I was nicotine's bitch for thirty years. It took a *lot* to quit listening to that mental screaming. I haven't won the fight against all my bugbears yet, but am knocking them off little by little. I have seen behind the veil a few times, and realise there is more to this life (by paradoxically being way less). I choose to face it and accept it, and thrive best I can. I don't want to be all about comfort. I want to remain connected with the animal in me, with my true nature. It is there where I find my strength and my best experience of life.'

Halfway through our Zoom conversation, Johnnie presses his face against his phone and points to his chin: instinctively I peer more closely, not quite sure what I'm looking at. 'Frostbite,' he announces and we both flinch back from our phone screens, instinctively reacting to the sudden proximity, even though we are physically thousands of miles apart. Is that the only part of his body that gets affected by the cold, I wonder, still trying to work out whether to ask him how he manages to slide so elegantly into a chest freezer wearing nothing but a tiny pair of Speedos.

For a moment, we are both silent, as if a boundary has been crossed. How does Johnnie feel about his body? I find him really expressive, in his facial expressions, body language and style of dressing, or undressing in the case of Speedos in sub-20° Fahrenheit. 'What I do is really physical most of the time, either when I'm climbing into my chest freezer, going from intense summer temperatures to intense cold, or when I'm dragging my sled out of the truck, loading it with equipment, hauling it across the lake to where I cut out my ice hole every winter. It's demanding on my body and mind because some days I just don't want to put in the work.'

Is he in touch with his physical self? 'Well, I'm not body shy any more, not like I used to be. I was never comfortable with my body when I was younger, so tall and skinny. But now, as I'm getting older, I see so many men with a paunch, I don't feel so bad about it. And yes, filming myself every time I climb into my freezer or the ice hole has helped hugely to desensitise me. You know, body confidence is every bit as relevant for men as it is for women. We get labelled like women do. I have been challenged by body image, and by how others perceive me (informed by the trauma of growing up misunderstood, labelled, and physically and mentally beaten for being different). I'm not gay, but I live in a small town, my clothes are different to other men's because I make a lot of them myself, I like colour and patterns. I don't want to blend in, I'm creative, musical … bizarrely, I feel accepted for who I am when I'm in the cold water. No one judges me for how I look, only what I do. It's very liberating and I can be truly me. The minimalist suits I wear are first and foremost a *very* practical effective piece of kit, in so many ways. But they are fun and a serious challenge, especially here in rural America.

'I would *love* to skinny dip,' comments Johnnie wistfully, 'and do any chance I get, but it is far too cold – dangerously, damagingly cold – to do so. Hands and feet aren't the only appendages the body shunts blood to. That penis gets so cold. Very painful. And nerve damage. Yeah, *not good*! I deal with the fingers and toes getting numb and shedding skin, but I draw the line in the swimsuit area! I had a scare last year, and am now more careful. Keep the damn wind off of it too, please!

'And that is my main reason for dipping: self-empowerment. I'm not a control freak, but knowing that my mind is a tool, which I am in charge of, is important in so much of my life. Cold will not control me. No fear of winter, of cold water, or of "discomfort". I am energised when I survive, when I remain connected to my desire.'

What originally drew me to Johnnie's story were the images of windswept, frozen wastelands, sun striking bizarre ice sculptures deliberately arranged around a dark pool of water in this icy landscape. A Christmas tree stands to one side, alone in its greenness and lushness. Everything else is white and cold. It makes you shiver just thinking about how quickly the strong winds would strip you of any residual body heat as you climbed up your ladder out of the ice hole. And yet, he survives and thrives on this extreme activity.

'When the water is a good few degrees warmer than the air, you get a false sense of warm; it is almost a relief to climb down into the water. And then you realise that the water is actually sucking the heat out of you really fast. And the wind chill finishes the job of freezing you unless you are prepared and move really fast and keep moving.' There are times when Johnnie comes out of the water on such a high that he feels all powerful, tempted to stand around and look at the place he has created. He has to force himself to act fast before his hands freeze and he won't be able to dress himself. Things would go rapidly downhill if that happened. He has to work at the mental game his mind is playing with his body.

Jonna Jinton, an artist, musician and filmmaker who lives in the woods in the far north of Sweden, initially inspired him to try ice bathing because her aesthetically stunning YouTube videos took all sense of danger and fear away from immersing yourself in ice, something all children are taught is dangerous. 'I envied her ice saw and wanted one,' he tells me. So he bought one and the next time he was at a friend's cabin, going from sauna to lake, he cut a hole in the ice for fun to see how his saw worked. The following morning as they were packing up to leave, he realised he'd left his ladder in the ice hole. The air temperature was 0 °C, but it was a peaceful, still morning, so he stripped off and calmly climbed down into the water. That's when he realised that it was something he wanted to have in his life on a regular basis.

The house he now lives in is the house where he was born. Although he has lived in many other places in the United States, nowhere else has kept drawing him back. There is a rootedness about the landscape, the people and the history that he has never experienced anywhere else. Other places may be more beautiful or dramatic, but somehow don't have gravity or roots. On the border between the Big Forest and the Prairies, the landscape is a criss-cross of lakes and rivers, trees and vast openness. Here, he is never more than five minutes from water; it is known as the land of 10,000 lakes and there are actually far more than that. I ask him what is so special about the place and his voice cracks slightly with emotion: 'the rich dark soil, trees, deep roots and the core of American history. This is the land of the Native Americans, the land white man saw and wanted and took, only 140 years ago, with violence and greed. They called it the Indian Uprising! But in truth it was just a massacre and the blood that was spilt was only Native American. I grew up being taught a certain way of thinking about it all, but I've explored it, questioned the books and want to continue to learn about their culture.'

Johnnie has always practiced yoga and explored Eastern religion, but since he has found cold water and ice, he finds himself more and more drawn to Native American imageries. As he drags his sled from his car to the place with the Christmas tree and the ice hole he has created, his muscles strain, his mind wanders and his heart fills with passion and longing to connect with those people who were there hundreds of years before him, living on and close to this lake all year round, dependent on it for their survival and deeply respectful of how quickly it could kill them, especially during the intense cold of the long winters.

These people grew up and lived on these rivers and lakes, got wet, must have got really cold and had no sauna to sit in to warm up, or change of clothes in their car. How did they cope with it? How did they have the mental strength to keep going? The connection to the water is deep, for them and for him. Sometimes when he is canoeing in the summer on a lake and sees a deer, he realises that although it's not the selfsame deer, it is the same deer that has been here for centuries. By visiting the same lake repeatedly, as the groups of Native Americans must have done, he feels he goes back in time and becomes part of history himself. And as he steps down his ladder into the cold water, he is celebrating that connection and that history in the knowledge that he does this out of choice, not necessity. It is a humbling experience.

I remember talking with Johnnie at one point and asking him whether he had ever considered he had a relationship with the lake as his soulmate. It had got him thinking about his whole experience in the town he had known all his life: 'It is so easy to live life by default; I live the majority of my experience that way. But now, with the lake anyway, it is different. I keep in mind the lifelong accumulation of experiences I have had there, the things I have learnt, so much time spent with friends, time alone. I choose to honour that and come with gratitude for our being able to know and express each other through our interaction.'

As Johnnie described how his feelings towards the lake he has known all his life had changed, I realised that our conversation had closed one door for him and opened another. Now familiarity had become anticipation and surprise. He never knows what he will find when he visits. Everything from the parking to the ice hole is different every day, with infinite variables combining to offer him an ever-changing perspective. When he arrives, he immediately begins taking in the changes: drifted snow, ice thickness, light, mysterious footprints. It is all there, alive, right now waiting, changing.

I felt physically exhausted after he went through how much work is involved in going out there every day to prepare that ice hole. This year there has been an almost constant wind, so he has had to shovel the whole place out every time he arrives. Then there's the cutting of the ice, breaking up the slabs and hauling the pieces out to the perimeter. 'The saw-cutting of the ice feels so very primitive to me. Something of a spear, or a harpoon. It really does feel like something of a harvest. I suppose sometime in the past I saw an old black-and-white movie, *Nanook of the North* maybe, of Eskimos with long spears cutting whale blubber into hunks and hauling it away. My saw plunges deeply in and out of the ice and cuts smoothly. Using my gloved hands or ice tongs, I drag the pieces out of the hole and then carry them away, water and slush coating my pants like blood and guts from the slaughter. Every day I reopen this wound in the lake, placing the shards around the hole and me for protection, for beauty, to warn of the fragile wound at the centre. It often takes me two hours until I am back in my car.'

Jack London is one of his favourite authors and his stories of trappers in Northern Alaska, always falling into streams and rivers, getting soaking wet, all speak of survival and discomfort. Johnnie recently fell into his own ice hole and instead of being scared or panicking, he had laughed. 'It's happening,' he thought as he stepped on to what he thought was the edge of the hole, but snow had drifted across in the night, so he fell straight down into the water. The air temperature was -14 °C and it was snowing. These were the conditions that Native Americans endured on a daily basis, so he could too. He rolled out of the hole, his body was still warm enough, and he continued to shovel for an hour and a half until he had cleared the snow away from the hole.

'I was only a few hundred yards away from my car, so I wasn't going to die!' he laughs loudly, which reminds me to ask him about his freezer and why he had decided to install one in his back yard for summer use only. 'Well, Wim Hof? I'm not one,' he says emphatically.

Wim Hof's teaching is quite antithetical to Johnnie's experience in the freezer or his ice hole. Having watched his videos where he raises the lid of the freezer and then slowly climbs in, one leg after the other, I can see that it is a controlled process. And he describes it as a meditation, an observation where his body does what it wants to do, but at the same time he is very conscious of what it is doing. He inhales slowly and deeply as he climbs in and then exhales as he moves down into the water in one fluid movement. He notices where the tension is in his mind and body, thinks about it and then pushes down on it until it relaxes and dissipates.

I ask him what he thinks about those who jump into a lake or even ice hole, almost making a joke out of the Zen moment of immersion. He loves how other bathers describe this way of entering the water as a lightning transition, an immediate burst of euphoria and energy. One of the fastest transitions you could possibly achieve, but clearly going against all the usual advice about not jumping into cold water. It feels odd to him unless it is in the context of the sauna–cold-dip–sauna experience he is used to. He wants to work with the sympathetic and parasympathetic nervous systems with a vision of being better able to control both at any given moment. The violent splashing movement, sound and feel of jumping in would not close down all other thought in the way that slow, silent, stealthy slipping like an aquatic creature does. He feels part of the water, not working against it. And he is yet another cold-water swimmer who describes how horrible taking a cold shower feels, how shocking, but not in a joyous way. For him, it provides neither pleasure nor pain, just distress and discomfort, but not something he can work with and turn around to a positive.

The vulnerability he has experienced while sitting in his ice hole alone in the dark is important to him because it has taught him about how to deal with feeling vulnerable and alone in other aspects of his life. His single state sometimes bothers him because of that same sense of vulnerability: you're fine until something goes wrong and then there is no one there to help you. But as he becomes more and more confident in being who he really is, he finds it harder and harder to find the connection he is searching for in a partner. Women might find him physically attractive, which is wonderful, but he needs them to look beyond that, to accept his creative spirit, the one that sews and puts together zany outfits, coordinates and choreographs solo ice baths during a blizzard and educates himself on alternative beliefs and cultures.

There is vulnerability on another level too in his lake: in the summer he can see the vegetation and snails that live on the bottom, he knows what is in the water with him; but in winter the water looks so much darker and is limited to the size of his ice hole. When he's sitting in that space, his mind tells him that there is a whole lake around him and anything could be in the water, creeping up on him from under the layer of ice. Even as he is slowly moving down into the water from his ladder, he tells himself it is the same bottom of the lake in winter as in summer, there is nothing new that only lurks there in winter. This fear is unwelcome and takes energy to subdue and control.

'I love to feel high on life, to feel connected to a bigger community beyond this borderlands town, although it is where my spirit is rooted. I love what my body is able to do and feel myself grow stronger physically and mentally. But I love the quiet moments where all thought closes down and it's just me and the cold.' Listening to Johnnie, I realise that every cold plunge does a similar thing for me too. It shuts down all automatic thinking (it can for some people anyway), and if I am quiet and mindful I can leave the water with a very refreshed outlook. It is a powerful reset for me.

Johnnie continues: 'I remember one time when I took a pretty serious psilocybin trip.[8] It was in the wintertime and I had planned this whole day because it was going to be a good ten hours probably. I brought blankets and sleeping bags and food and extra clothing and all this stuff.

'I had taken the medicine and was definitely under the effects and I got to my place and was setting up and at some point I was going through my bags and pulling things out to get set up and I realised that this "other me" had made all these things and planned out and prepared for "future me". It's kind of hard to describe, but I was so deeply touched that this other part of me loved and cared for me enough to think of every detail that I would need on this experience to be safe and comfortable. Does that make sense? It was really a powerful moment and teacher of self-love. And now when I am thinking about it, it is something that I can be aware of when I'm out there on the ice (or anytime). It's a way to look at self-love, which isn't always very easy for me at all.'

I've never explored psilocybin-assisted therapy, but after talking with Johnnie I googled it and was fascinated to discover that it is where the 'default mode network' in our brain gets shut down. This is all the automatic thinking and processing we do, where the mind doesn't really see or hear what's before us, but tells us what everything is because of past experience. It 'knows' all this already. Johnnie's words echoed in my mind as I started to transcribe our conversation, 'It is also all the rumination, the repeating of story over and over ... our thoughts become our tracks down a sledding hill. Fresh tracks eventually cross and we follow our earlier trail. Then it becomes a rut, a bobsled run we can't jump out of. The psilocybin is like a blanket of fresh snow on that hillside, allowing us to make new paths, form new thoughts, see things differently. We can just slip into the same groove

8   Psilocybin is a naturally occurring psychedelic prodrug compound produced by more than 200 species of fungi, more commonly known as 'magic mushrooms'. Although illegal in the UK and some other countries, psilocybin has become popular worldwide, with increasing scientific evidence that microdosing, where you ingest microscopic amounts, can be beneficial to those suffering from depression and other mental health issues. In parts of North America, psilocybin is legal.

again, but if we are mindful and deliberate, we can change our thoughts, become unhooked from trauma, and unleash creativity.'

Another powerful thing I've heard other cold-water swimmers talk about is just how the cold slows you down, brings your focus down to a level so much smaller, and this is how Johnnie describes this process: 'I am observing and appreciating very small and fleeting things – bubbles, ice crystals, snails caught in the ice, snow drifts, even the wind. It re-minds me, shows me my own fleeting, temporary nature, demonstrates what a crazy experience it is to live with this body machine which does all this ice cutting and lifting, temperature regulation, shedding and replacing of skin which I freeze off. The hilarity of extreme body part shrinking!'

I sense we may be straying back on to the path of tiny Speedos, but I understand Johnnie a bit better now and easily get how his creativity is sparked out there and how he feels he is back to being a little kid building a snow fort and how it is a distraction, definitely, and for a while you are not thinking of other issues in your life. 'I only respond to the ice, the shapes, the light and it all sort of tells me where it wants to go. Then I undress and slip down into the middle of it all. Just me the observer.'

And the muskrat, I add. Johnnie's laugh echoes across the Atlantic. He's already told me about his friend the muskrat (a sort of small beaver), who watches him while he is sitting in his ice hole, waiting until he is done, and then scuttles across, dives in and pulls out strands of vegetation, sparse in winter, but tickly enough to bother Johnnie.

Perhaps the last thing, maybe odd but worth mentioning, is all the planning and preparation and execution that Johnnie loves to do. It is the opposite of so much of what he has already explained to me, yet it is a bone to throw his mind to keep it happy. There is a process, the gear and the game, to make the activity go smoothly and safely. 'Someone DOES have to watch out for me while I am doing this. Make decisions, coordinate movements and problem-solve.'

FIEN

Fien lives in Belgium and has been a cold-water swimmer for a few years, initially in the sea, but now she has also started using a chest freezer so that she can have easy access to cold water. In Belgium it is illegal to swim not only in the sea but in all public waters (rivers, lakes) without a guard. This is also the case in the Ardennes where Fien sometimes goes. The sea is only three kilometres away from her, but isn't always an option because of storms, currents and strong winds. The only clubs are in Bruges. But they only meet once or twice a week and you have to be a member and some of the clubs demand that you wear a wetsuit.

'Your breasts and vagina are the most difficult parts of your body when you go in the freezer,' she says, wincing as she lifts her other leg up and into her chest freezer and plants both feet on the bottom, her hands holding on to the sides. 'I don't need to breathe any more to do this, although I do it because it feels good. I can control the pain of the cold, a bit like childbirth.' From my warm study, I wince in empathy as I watch her on our video chat. Her chest freezer sits on a wooden platform under a treehouse. There is a willow tree that she was given when she got married and it creates a bit of privacy from the road that passes her garden. While she is sitting calmly in her freezer, we both hear the sound of horses trotting along the road. 'The fishermen coming back from the sea,' she explains.

Fien looks so relaxed and comfortable, up to her chin in transparent water, with broken ice floating around her shoulders. Now and again, she stirs the ice around with her bare hands and grins at the camera. She knows it's cold, but doesn't feel it as cold any more. I've watched her climb into the chest freezer, splash her face and the back of her neck and then sink lower and lower, the control evident in every flicker of pleasure at the corners of her mouth, her eyes open and watching me and then looking into the freezer itself.

I'm intrigued to know how she operates the freezer, how she stops it from going mouldy. I have a Japanese bathtub, all wood, which I can heat with a wood burner, but I mostly leave it cold. I've found that it is extremely easy to maintain, with no need for a filter or any additions to the water. I just make sure I am clean every time I go in it and maybe empty it every couple of months, add a tiny bit of bleach and scrub it thoroughly to prevent any sliminess or blackening of the interior. Then I refill it to the brim and put the lid back on. Fien has a similar routine, only she has had to put silicone around the outlet so that water doesn't seep out of the freezer and rework itself back through, potentially bringing chemicals into the water. The timer to refreeze is on now and again to maintain a cold temperature, but if it was on permanently there would be no water, just a block of ice. Plus, like me, she is careful to ensure she doesn't bring any outside debris into the water, so, as she has to cross her garden and there is lawn, she wipes her feet on a piece of plastic carpet next to the freezer itself.

'Oh, and I have to remind myself to unplug it before I climb in!' Something I'd probably forget to do, I think!

Why does she use a freezer, though? It's simple, she tells me. The sea is not that close and Belgium has some strange laws about swimming in the sea. You're not allowed to go without lifeguards and there are often people ready to call the police if they see you. You never know who might feel like calling the police, so you are always slightly on edge. That's why she often swims near the windsurfers, because she is less obvious to anyone watching, but there is a risk of being surfed over! During lockdown the police used drones to monitor people on the beach: you were permitted to walk, move, but not sit and have a drink or play on the beach, so although it was possible, it was not a relaxing experience.

With the freezer in her garden she is free to bathe whenever she feels the need. For physical and emotional pain, whichever she is experiencing the most, sometimes both. Physical pain as a result of long Covid is exhausting and this draining of energy has stolen her innate playful nature. She grieves for who she once was and hopes that one day she can become that person again. In the meantime, she reconnects to whatever Fien is left: in the freezer she finds calm and peace, in the stormy waves of the sea she is uplifted and recognises the animal passion she once took for granted.

As a lone swimmer, with no need to swim with a pack, Fien accepts the risks – in fact, she embraces the discomfort that the touch of the cold water inflicts on her aching and pain-ridden body. No neoprene whatsoever, however cold the water. She no longer feels the cold and can't decide whether that is because she is so used to it now, with taking a cold shower every morning. She explains that she has always loved water, even before suffering with long Covid. The cold water is a tool in her healing, but healing is not the main reason; but rather playfulness, freedom, nature, mindset, a kick in the arse and the feeling that everything is possible if she can manage the cold water.

In the freezer, even when it is close to 1 °C, all she feels is pleasure as the cold bites into her. It is odd, she says, because she has no problems with her feet or hands in the freezer, only when she bathes in nature, the sea or rivers and lakes. And brain freeze? What's that? she laughs. Even in a fierce winter sea with waves crashing over her head, all she feels is exhilaration, not cold. The only problem she's ever had is when she was in the Ardennes and there was snow. When she came out of the water it felt as if she was walking on blocks of ice, but once she'd got her sheeplined boots on, the feeling came back and she was fine.

By now, Fien has stepped out of her freezer and is sitting at a garden table chatting to me: swimsuit and jumper, no after-drop, no need for a hot drink. 'How I have changed since I've been a cold-water swimmer! Four years ago if I'd imagined sitting in my garden in winter like this, pah! Give me my thermal underwear, two pullovers and a shawl, scarf, jacket, blanket and I'd still be cold. Maybe my circulation has improved?'

Could it be the menopause? I ask. Our metabolism changes along with our hormone levels, so we can tolerate the cold better, or actually seek out the cold to calm hot flushes and irritability!

'Maybe … one thing I know for sure is my skin tone has improved; my breasts feel lifted and everything feels younger! How is that?' Fien's laugh is infectious. We share a similar sense of the ridiculous and slightly naughty, two qualities that can be so fragile as you grow older and have experienced bad relationships where your sense of self-worth takes a pounding.

Nothing can stop you from being who you are, though, and the thoughts that you have about your need for love and physical connection. If there's one thing cold-water swimming always gives back to me, and I could talk about this for hours with Fien, it is a sense of play and desire to be playful. When pain, emotional or physical, is overriding, it becomes impossible to be yourself, that side of you becomes crushed. Solo ice bathing liberates your mind and reconnects you to your body: you are acutely aware of every inch of skin, every hair follicle and every subtle change in how you feel. Once you have defrosted, those feelings of being fully alive and physically awake don't disappear just like that. It feels as if you are in a state of arousal, not just sexual, but soulful. As nature intended you to be. Before life thundered through your core and ripped away primal thoughts and feelings.

Fien echoes my thoughts with ones of her own, which speak of learning to trust herself, to not accept second best and to live her life as truthfully as possible. The concentration she applies to dunking in her freezer carries through to so many other things: working from home, restoring her energy, caring for her two sons and reinventing fashion. But she is weak too. Her passionate nature means even if she knows she should rest for the day, if she has the urge to drive to the Ardennes and be in the forests, she will pack up the van and go. And then need to rest for two extra days.

'I was brought up by photographers: my mum and dad ran a photography shop and we lived above it. At night, I used to sometimes hear burglars breaking in, but I learnt not to panic. I would open my window, shout out to frighten them and wake my parents and everyone in the neighbourhood. The adrenaline of my fear must have made me act rather than just hide and stay quiet. But I didn't feel any panic, not once. Maybe that ability to calm myself to the point of not feeling anything at all has become a coping mechanism in any stressful event in life, including very cold water?'

But how do you feel when you are in moving water? I am curious to know whether this rigid control she has over herself can be broken by a different type of water to the icy depths of her chest freezer. I seem to have struck a chord, because her eyes light up and her voice sounds excited. 'Yes! The sea or a river, they are moving bodies of water, it flows, moves, rushes and pushes. It is in control of me and I love that sense of abandoning myself to whatever it wants to do with me. I feel my spirit leaping out of my body, celebrating being alive, being strong and having the power to play with the waves or the current.'

She's right, you can't control the sea or a river, and maybe it is that sense of relief from allowing yourself to lose control that takes us back to our true selves, strips us bare and reveals what we really are. By braving the cold water and trusting it to bring us back to ourselves, we are opening the door to opportunity and liberation.

THE
THINKER

A Thinker sees both sides of a situation, isn't afraid to talk about the negative aspects and is always ready to help resolve them. However, an overthinker spends a lot of time worrying about what might happen and feels uncomfortable throwing caution to the wind and trying new things. Usually risk-averse, Thinkers weigh up a situation and look for possible things that can go wrong. On the flip side, once a Thinker has made a decision, they will stick to it.

JAY

Jay is Canadian, but has ended up living in Norway. His house is right on the ocean and his cold-water journey started here from his own floating dock. In his previous life he spent years in the wilderness of various parts of Canada, trapping and hunting for pleasure and it was also how he earned a living. No stranger to physical discomfort, he has taken to the icy waters of Norwegian fjords with relish and gratitude. His daily ice baths started when the Covid-19 pandemic hit Norway and he has committed to a daily ice bath ever since.

'Step on the yellow crate and sit down on any part of that,' suggested Jay, pointing to the rim of a huge oak barrel, which he built himself. 'Bring your feet up on to the edge, kind of scooch around, scoochy scoochy, put your feet down and use your arms to support yourself. You're tall enough to do that. There you go.'

The sound of water spilling out of the barrel as I displaced it was deafening and peculiarly satisfying. I found I was talking to myself, 'Squat. Okay. Breathing.'

Then Jay's voice came back into focus, 'You can lean on the edge as you're squatting down, makes it easier to cross your heels behind you.'

'I can't cross my heels or bend my legs that much', I groaned. But, after a lot of scrunching and wriggling I had settled down into the water and took a moment to look at where I was. Right on the edge of a Norwegian river/fjord, with a wooden floating jetty in front of me, a handful of boats moored up safely, protected from winter storms, but prone to filling with snow. Across the river was the island of Hisøy, a beautiful place where rich Oslo people come for a couple of weeks each year to enjoy their 'summer' homes.

That night, there were enough lights in the windows to create electric beauty and watery reflections. I felt I would have been content to observe this view for hours on end, because it was in a constant state of flicker and waft. The view from the jetty to downtown Arendal had brought tears to my eyes on the first morning I stood there. I couldn't actually believe I was there, in Norway, doing what I was doing. Bizarrely, I felt my mother's presence in this place and I still don't understand why.

We'd put a jar of lights in the barrel and I rolled it around because the lights kept flickering on and off: a loose connection and also a bit of a distraction from the intense cold of the water that gripped my shoulders and sent shock waves up my neck into my brain.

'So, the point of that tub is the stillness. There's no sand, no rocks, no weeds, no waves, there's you and perfectly still, perfectly cold water,' explained Jay.

To be honest, it felt like my tub, but because movement in it was more restricted I also almost felt trapped in the cold physically and perhaps psychologically. After several barrel sessions I began to feel more comfortable about the dimensions and could relate to what Jay described as 'being held in stillness', which to him is a comforting rather than constraining feeling.

'I spent years looking out of the window of my house and hating everything that I saw. Everything that I didn't have and couldn't have, and everything I had to find time and energy and money to do. It wasn't until I started doing this and spending my time down here that I had found peace and quiet because the cold made the screeching noise in my head go away and I started to see how beautiful it can be: in the sunshine because it's south-facing, but especially at night, when all the lights on the houses are shining on the water. I spent a good chunk of the summer reminding myself every morning, if it wasn't raining, no matter if it was cold or windy, to take my cacao down to the end of the dock and sit in my red chair. There I'd reflect on how my thoughts and views on it for so many years didn't have to be my thoughts for the rest of my life. That was a big deal.'

Jay built his barrel in a friend's workshop during summer 2020. It fits his dimensions perfectly. In order to sit and crouch, the barrel is larger in diameter than the length of his thigh bone. He worked out the measurement from knees to shoulder precisely so he would be up to his neck in water. The important thing about it is that it's still and cold – in summer he can refill it from the garden hose daily and have 12° groundwater, which is colder than the ocean.

'In summer, the ocean here is too warm, as high as 20–22°, and has hundreds of jellyfish. By the end of May, I abandon the ocean and go to streams, or use the barrel. No natural supply of regular, repeatable, reliable cold water.' For Jay, if it's not 12° or colder then he's not getting the 'physical, mental, emotional release. That is the point of it for me.'

I felt we needed to backtrack a little, to why, when and where he started his ice bathing. I knew he had made it his mission to dip 'every damn day', but I was curious to know more about this commitment and what would happen if he missed a day.

It started in March 2020 when the world started to shut down in the face of Covid-19. Many Norwegians were incredulous that their lives would be affected, so when it was clear things were going to change and a type of low-level fear crept into the school playground, Jay took his two children down to his dock one morning and told them there was no need to be afraid of the virus – fear doesn't need to stop us from doing hard things. He had a lot of personal stuff going on, but mostly was concerned about the kids and the idea that they would talk about this time in their cohort for the rest of their lives. He didn't want them to grow up with the idea that you had to run and hide in fear. 'Part of me wanted to protect them from my own experience because that's what I had been doing for a whole bunch of years and I've been unable to fix my own issues.'

He did some background research on ice bathing, understood the benefits, but hadn't really thought much about them. He just wanted his kids to see that he could do something that was really hard and he wasn't going to die. Even though it took work and willpower, he could do it and be happy about it. The dominant thought at the time was you didn't have to live in fear. He took them every day, at some point in the morning, but there was no schedule. Three minutes was the minimum he wanted to be able to stay in and he remembers climbing down the ladder into the 4° water, the cold, burning, tingling, which was so painful in the beginning while he was learning, his body adjusting and becoming comfortable with or accustomed to the discomfort.

'There was a riot going on in my brain and body, the kids were firing a thousand typical kid questions, along with handfuls of snow to make the water colder! "Just give Daddy a few seconds, let me catch my breath." And I haven't missed a day since.'[9]

'The cold water brings clarity. For most of my adult life I have had what I call a noisy head, a lot of thoughts, voices, chatter, not multiple personality voices, but I hear my thoughts and I have a lot of them because I am interested in a lot of different topics. I found that generally, after the huffing and puffing, within the first minute in good cold water I had regained physical control and then the quiet and peace in my brain. That was quite exciting because I didn't have that ever once I was in Norway.'

Do I ever have silence in my head? I asked myself. Rarely. I know what Jay means about hearing his thoughts. The inside of my head is playing out so many different scenarios most of the time and I'm sure it even does this when I'm asleep because often I wake up knowing how to resolve an issue, or how to write a paragraph in a book.

But, never mind me, what did Jay mean by 'good cold water'?

'I really like 5°. It's the first temperature where when I get in, my body is like "holy shit, this is cold" – plus it was 5° when I started dipping off my wharf. Growing up in Canada, I knew you didn't want to be in the water, especially if the water is cold. There's a causal relationship: if you fall in the water, you die in the winter. I know people who have. You actively do things to avoid falling in water, which is bizarre considering everyone drives trucks on ice and goes ice fishing. Winter is long and cold in Canada and when you fly over that part of Canada you'll see a million tiny freshwater lakes. We naturally use that, and it sounds terrifying or appalling to people who don't grow up in that environment: like the time I was ice fishing and my dad walked out to see how I was getting on. I could feel the ice flexing under his feet, it was so thin – I shouted at him to not get any closer. And the first time you're in a truck and drive across the ice road

9   At the time of publication (November 2022) it has been nearly 1,000 consecutive days.

to the three-way stop, with stop signs. Now that blows a lot of people's minds. But it's normal if that's how you grow up.'

I saw something interesting here: someone who has a lifetime's experience of knowing cold, but also an inbuilt urge to keep out of cold water because he knows it could kill him. To make that transition from childhood fear and caution to embracing something that can kill you must have required a motivation of steel.

Over the first summer, Jay found that his main motivation for his daily dip had changed. He had started to clue in to the benefits he was experiencing, especially in a mental sense. 'Selfish' is a word he used a lot when he described his commitment to himself on a daily basis, but he knew he was getting this peace and that was a big deal, something he hadn't had in so long and hadn't realised how sorely he needed it in his life. So he kept going.

And what would happen if you took a day off? I asked. I thought I already knew the answer, but wanted to give Jay the opportunity to explore his own psyche and motivation. 'If I take a day off, maybe it'll unwind,' he said. 'And that brings a whole new fear! Maybe it'll all go away and I'll have to go back to the beginning to get that kind of peace back. So I have to keep going. It's non-negotiable.'

Personal resilience has been spoken about by many of the people I've talked to and I would agree that if you can be brave enough to step into cold water, you have more chance of being brave enough to face other obstacles in life. But for Jay the reprieve and peaceful silence he experiences during his dip go hand in hand with a stronger mental resilience that spills over into real-life pedestrian situations.

Was it coming to Norway that set off that lower resilience? 'Yes, the relocation most definitely overwhelmed me in so many ways. I lost all of my ability to deal with things; all of my resilience and that spiralled and caused all sorts of other problems. I'd always been a resourceful person, able to think outside the box, a creative problem-solver. My parents had brought me up to be capable, so I can do, not necessarily well, a lot of things: build houses, rig explosives ... I would love to dynamite a hole in the ice. Nothing puts the lead in your pants like blowing stuff up.' I wanted to dare Jay to try this out, but the legal and environmental ramifications have confined it to the realms of fantasy (for the time being).

'Coming here, I had to relearn everything. I love travelling and experiencing different cultures, but I felt like I needed to fit in and everything was so different and confusing. I had nowhere to start fitting in or to build to the next thing. Everybody else in my life was thinking this is the most amazing country ever, so what's your problem? I was left on my own to figure it out. But I didn't. I didn't want to leave the house. I just felt weird and disconnected. Judged. If I was with the kids in the grocery store, I didn't want anyone to hear me talking in English, to be obviously a foreigner. If I don't open my mouth you wouldn't know because I almost look Norwegian.'

Certainly Scandinavian, with his height, fair hair and complexion, blue eyes and seemingly reserved and quiet nature. Loud music playing on his jetty while he dived in again and again completely confirmed that he is far more than first appearances – a man of many layers who is willing to peel them back, however painful, to reach the part of himself he was scared he had lost.

I used this opportunity to ask Jay about body confidence and how he thought daily cold-water immersion had improved his own or whether it hadn't ever been an issue for him. By filming ourselves and posting on social media, we all get the opportunity to look at our bodies and be hypercritical or learn to embrace how amazing they are to adapt to the cold water as often as we expect them to. Men as well as women have those 'bits' they hate, so how did Jay feel about his body now after nearly two years of stripping down to skimpy swim trunks? What did he see when he looks in the mirror?

'Only since living in Norway have I begun to think "yuck" – even though I hadn't put on any weight or lost muscle, it didn't change the fact that I would see myself and think "yuck". Then, suddenly, I had a mind shift and saw beauty and strength in my body. Here you are, I thought, and I just haven't appreciated you for as long as I can remember. One morning after my dip, I looked at myself in the mirror and actually felt "virile" for the first time in years! The man I wanted to be.'

This is what I wanted to hear: a man in his early fifties describing how he still had fire in his belly. Confirmation that it's not just a female prerogative to want to feel amazing, strong and desirable in their later years, to regain their self-confidence. Men can aspire to have 'it' too.

'The biologist in me often steps in,' laughed Jay, 'I end up examining my body for signs of change due to the cold water, or I deliberately stay in longer to see how my body reacts.'

Jay started to take his body temperature from around January 2021 until March that year. It was a severe winter and from his records he knows that for more than fifty consecutive days he had hypothermia with an average core temperature close to 31.2 °C. He paid attention to the temperature of the water, time in the water and core temperature fifteen minutes after getting out of the water. He was interested in how his body reacted, not how he felt mentally at that point. He knew already that it was how he felt when he came to the water that dictated how he would feel on leaving it. He recalled a day when he had just added water to his barrel rather than emptying it as was his usual practice to keep it at its coldest. So the water was maybe 15 °C, but after only a minute or so of sitting in it he was shaking and shivering so hard that the water was splashing out of the barrel. He'd thought to himself, 'It's not even cold, it's a frigging bathtub in here and I'm shaking like a madman.' He puts this reaction down solely to his poor mental and emotional state when he climbed in the barrel, with a cacophony of difficult issues all hitting him at the same time in his personal life.

Conversely, there have been days where the water was 1 °C (he did a ten-minute Live chat at 0°) and he'd jumped in off his dock, or climbed down the ladder and all he'd had to do was take a breath, a few deep breaths and he was calm: physically and mentally.

The only time Jay feels anything like physical panic, where his body says, 'this is cold, this is a problem, we are losing heat faster than we can deal with, you need to do something about it' – is when the water is moving as it is at a local waterfall. Here, if there is snow melt, the water can be around 1–2° maximum and is moving fast and hard. It's a tricky place to get into when there's a lot of water and he has to sit in a weird position where his backside is floating in air, but his feet are braced against rocks in front of him.

The water pounds down on to his head and shoulders. The physical panic coursing through his body fascinates him. It is as if his body is shouting at his brain, 'We're going to die!'

'I know we're not going to die, but I can feel the heat being stripped out of my body at such a rate that I know that it's out of proportion. I've had enough days dipping to have experimented with hot drinks, warm water in a bucket and so on to know how best to warm up on any given day.'

So far, we've just discussed hanging off his ladder, kneeling in his barrel, crouching under a waterfall, but what about swimming? Just looking at the ocean he has at his fingertips makes me want to dive in and swim around. From his dock to his neighbour's must be around thirty metres, I reckoned, with a large red buoy in the middle – did he ever do lengths between the docks for fun? Had he ever considered doing some distance swimming, perhaps a winter swimming event?

'But I didn't know how to swim.' For someone who grew up on a lake and has spent most of his life working on or near water and boats, it's a difficult concept to grasp. Of course, he knew how to swim enough to save himself if he fell in the water, but actual swimming in any sustained fashion was anathema to him. Why would he want to do that? Of course, as his resilience to stress grew stronger, so did his determination to push himself out of his comfort zone. The thought of swimming from his dock to his neighbour's terrified him, because in his head he knew that if he got to the point where he couldn't swim any more, what would he do? Sink. Drown. It wasn't like running, where if you get out of breath you just stop, have a break and carry on. The first few swims across that terrifying, deep water were significant; he felt drained afterwards, not from the cold, but the mental effort required to keep swimming. He started in November 2020 and took baby steps in terms of distance.

Then, in the middle of October 2021, something arrived in the post that changed his life. Someone had been observing his progress and knew exactly what would help him reach his goal. The bright green tow float was something he knew existed, but he'd thought it was what really good swimmers used in events. It was something he didn't know he needed or that it was a device that would allow him to swim.

'It was mind-blowing. I'd go swimming and get to the point where I'd think, I can't go any further, I'm too tired, cold or have run out of breath. First, I'd tell myself to keep going, then get to the point where I knew I was going to sink, so I'd roll over and grab the float. Obviously there was some danger in that, but it was amazing how when I thought, I'm done, I'm going to drown now, I'd mark that distance in my mind and keep going with the knowledge that when I actually start to sink, I'll just grab the float. How much more swimming was possible because now I had a bail-out plan in a way I had never had one before: it had always been sink or swim.'

Given that he swam through some of the coldest months of the year, his transition is incredible. It would take him around fourteen minutes to swim 350 metres, which in water of around 2–3 °C is phenomenal. When he got out, he could feel that his skin didn't slide properly over his muscles, so that told him that the thin, not fascia or fat, but bubbly material between skin and muscles was pretty much frozen because it wouldn't slide any more.

'It's not a matter of will I dip or swim today, but when. If the sun's out I'll go in the morning, but if it's raining and shitty, I'll think to myself, let's just wait, if shitty I can have a dip at midnight when I know it's been shitty all day. But every day, never less than three minutes, my heart, the heat generator of my body, is underwater. Finding the coldest water available is part of the experience and stops me from getting bored with the relentless commitment I have undertaken.'

There have been a few rather atrocious nights where, because of the bizarre work life Jay has, it's close to midnight, it's pitch black, but he knows he's still got to do his dip.

'I realise that a half-arsed dip is not going to cut it. I have whatever is going on in my life at that specific moment and I know that "good cold water" is the only thing that will silence the noise in my head and "wash the shit of life away". That's a pretty accurate description. My dip is not a magic cure-all, but I am always happier and lighter of spirit. Many times it gives me a bit of bandwidth to then have perspective on what's going on in my life.

'Making myself enough of a priority to carve out time every day makes me, fact proven, a better person, for every person I interact with that day. But I'll freely admit that one of the greatest limiting factors to my daily dip is not always time, but fear. I'm not sure if I can pick out one single thing I'm afraid of, but I know how I feel as I prepare to meet the water, even during the summer months when my barrel is filled with ground temperature water, so in Norway that's around 13 °C. I stand looking at the water for long seconds in fear before I get in. Skin pebbled like the Thanksgiving turkey, nipples like diamonds, kneecaps bouncing like the needle on a sewing machine, I let that moment linger in my mind. Then imagination becomes reality. A small gasp, a long exhale and a smile.

'But I can't lie and tell you that facing every fear ends this way and I truly know the difference between facing emotional and physical fears, but I can tell you that in my life bliss has rarely come without fear first. I just hope that I'll always have the ability to see which fears are just blackout curtains blocking the sunshine, the joy, the love and the bliss that is on the other side and then draw them back, no matter how it chills my spine.'

JONNY

Jonny always wanted to live somewhere epic and has recently made the Lake District his home. A familiar face at Kendal Mountain Festival and Editor of *Outdoor Swimmer* magazine for over seven years, his passion for outdoor swimming of every kind is stronger than ever. He has swum throughout the year with absolutely no neoprene for over thirteen years and has participated in many cold-water swimming championships around the world.

'I'll say this once and then I'll have to kill you,' said Jonny as we sat in my car after our swim at Millerground in the Lake District, 'I believe a lot of cold-water swimmers are ex-clubbers and ravers.'

He laughed at my expression and explained what he meant. 'Chasing that high, the endorphin rush we used to get on an all-night dance floor.' Oh yes, I remember, my Wednesday-night sessions at the Camden Palace were clearly excellent training for cold-water swimming!

Jonny rewinds to the South London Swimming Club Christmas Day swim at Tooting Bec Lido, over a decade ago. Ann, a neighbour, had said, 'come down'. So Jonny did. It was 2 °C. He got in and got straight back out. Tooting Bec Lido is a really special place in which to have started his cold-water swimming journey, being the first place in the United Kingdom to host a swimming event, the inaugural UK Cold Water Swimming Championships (2006). Already a member of the South London Swimming Club, Jonny now put his winter membership to good use. This enabled him to swim right through the year and he soon realised he was part of a wonderful community of highly experienced and supportive cold-water swimmers. It also allowed use of the poolside sauna, a real asset when the lido was hovering around 2 °C.[10] Even though he'd already completed his first Great North Swim at the age of thirty when he had been looking for a way to get back into shape after years of neglecting his body (probably too much raving, I teased him), Jonny spent the next ten years or so building up his resilience to cold water, mostly at Tooting Bec Lido, but also by participating in a plethora of international ice-swimming championships – in Latvia, Poland, Finland, Sweden and Germany amongst others.

With an ice kilometre fingertips away from being under his belt, Jonny has pushed his swimming ability, but in his first winter in the Lakes, something has happened to his motivation. No longer craving the competitive edge that swimming distance brings, his focus has shifted to the experiential side of wild swimming. He often wants to be out in the lake on his own, especially during the summer after work. 'A dusk skinny dip with bats swooping down on my head, the Langdale Pikes tantalisingly close, yet so far away, gives me space to empty my head of the debris of so many huge changes over the last few years. I want peace and solitude: at that point the temperature of the water is insignificant; I just need to be immersed.'

But the cold undoubtedly adds another element, admitted Jonny, which he is highly sensitive to at certain times of the year. 'In summer, there is a moment, towards the middle of September, when I'm done with tepid water and I crave the bite of the cold. Conversely, by late March, early April, I'm starting to think, oh, for God's sake, I'm ready for some heat now.'

He also used to swim at the Royal London Docks, which was quite a long train journey across South London, but it gave him time to process his thoughts and he felt safe to do so because he knew at the Docks there was cold water waiting to receive his overthinking and release him from worries. It was as if his brain handed itself over to his body when it knew it wasn't in a good place, a form of self-medication. Conversely, thinks Jonny, if you're

10 So successful was the first UK Cold Water Swimming Championships that the Finnish Winter Swimming Team invited the South London Swimming Club (SLSC) to host the biannual World Winter Swimming Championships at Tooting Bec Lido in 2008. Now, although the World Championships go to different Eastern European countries every other year, the UK Championships is firmly fixed alternate years at Tooting. The Finns presented SLSC with a poolside sauna and two wood-fired hot tubs to say thank you for agreeing to host the event.

in a good place before you swim, the giddiness and the dancing around afterwards can escalate the rush of endorphins and serotonin. 'When I was younger, I danced all night with friends and strangers; there was a very real sense of community and connection – similar to the cold-water swimming community!'

And there is one community in particular that is close to Jonny's heart, here in the Lake District: the Blue Mind Men Community, which he has helped to set up. He invited me to join one of their Sunday-morning swims at Rayrigg, Windermere. 'It's not just for men, although primarily we want to give men a space that is different to their usual day-to-day environment. The kind of community that is caring, kind and supportive, one that invites you to leave the ego and macho persona in the car park.' He is adamant that Blue Mind Men can be anything its members want it to be, with no agenda, no formality apart from a five-minute opening circle where everyone says their name and a few words about how they have been feeling and what they are bringing to the water that day.

In the wake of a succession of winter storms, Windermere was amazingly placid, although there were white horses charging down the centre of the lake. The space between the two flooded jetties was an oasis of calm, grey, cold water. On the way down through the Central Lakes, I'd seen fallen trees left from the last storm and newly swollen becks and torrents crashing down the fellside to land on tarmac and create difficult driving conditions. Given these appalling conditions, it was surprising to see at least fifteen individuals arriving through the trees in silence, and then greeting each other slightly awkwardly on the lakeside and peering out at what they were about to swim in.

Once Jonny arrived, the mood changed and an air of anticipation wove the strangers together. We stripped off and wandered down to the water's edge, some taking slightly longer than others to wade into the water, but within minutes I found I was swimming with twelve men and three women, all grinning or grimacing, but all present and brave enough to show up for themselves and for each other. I was witness to a community in the making. I offered someone my neoprene gloves as I could see that she was holding her hands out of the water and therefore wasn't able to swim, just stand.

Our little community was doing something incredibly simple, but not easy. For a handful it was only the second time they'd been in the water, but to watch how their faces changed when they realised how good it felt is one of the best reasons to swim with a group like this. I need to be reminded sometimes how far I've come in my own cold-water journey by seeing others start theirs. How else can we appreciate what we expect our bodies and minds to endure and what better way to build up resilience in so many things? It's simple: bathe nearly naked in cold water!

Building resilience was the key to Jonny's escape from South London. During the third national lockdown he gave up alcohol and caffeine for six months, took daily cold showers and ran bare-chested round Crystal Palace Park in the dark, through some of the coldest nights we've seen in the UK for many years. 'Basically, I lived like a monk for six months,' said Jonny, 'only without the hair shirt!' It must have been tough to go out there on his own night after night, training his body to accept and deal with physical discomfort. But he laughed and said he actually really enjoyed it and believed it was a positive period of growth where he harnessed the power of the cold to achieve something special despite the constraints of the coronavirus pandemic.

'The more I built up my resistance, the better I felt. Everything toned up, not just my body, but my thinking, my planning ability, my motivation and my self-awareness. I knew that if I could turn myself into this person who was brave and strong enough to break through physical pain barriers like this, then I could be brave enough to break any ties I had left in London and pursue my dream of living somewhere extraordinary.' And so he did.

But, before moving to the Lake District, he had one last experience with city ice. Belair Park in Dulwich has a duck pond which had frozen over, a temptation too great for Jonny and a few of his friends. One Sunday morning, while only dog walkers were about, the sound of axes smashing through ice rang out across the pond. A feathery, goosy cold fix, accompanied by the soft 'ooooo' sounds of bodies receiving pleasure from intense cold. It was joyous because of how ridiculous it was and Jonny realised how far he'd travelled along the slippery road of being a cold-water swimmer: prepared to give almost anything a go if it flipped the switch.

Back to raving and clubbing, it seems, which brought me to ask Jonny whether he'd ever experienced the after-drop. As someone who knows how his body reacts to extreme physical effort, had he ever pushed himself beyond the beyond? 'Good question,' he responded, 'and not an easy one to answer … I have definitely pushed myself beyond my limits. One memorable time was at Beckenham Park Lake where I was swimming with a group in a professional capacity, so it's somewhat embarrassing, I suppose, but then again, maybe it's because I was so busy, so focused on other people that I ignored the cues my body was giving me. A valuable lesson.'

It was grossly unfair of him to leave me dangling like that, so I pressed him for detail. He is, after all, an experienced editor and journalist, so he knows the importance of detail! 'I needed a chill-out room, somewhere safe to sit until the feeling of not being with it had passed, but there wasn't even a sauna, which acts in the same way as a chill-out room. So I just sat and waited until I could remember how to put my underpants on.'

'Is that your barometer?' I asked Jonny, trying to keep a straight face.

'Exactly that,' he responded. 'You have to be able to look after yourself, especially if, like me, you want to swim alone. So you need to know yourself through and through. To do that, you have to have pushed yourself on a couple of occasions, met your limit and then pushed beyond that. But it's scary to stay in too long.'

But that fear has helped Jonny overcome extreme shyness, even as an adult, and helped him feel more sure of his place in the world. Without it he knows he would never have been Editor of *Outdoor Swimmer* magazine, sat on the Kendal Mountain Festival podium and talked in front of hundreds of Gore-Tex-clad outdoors enthusiasts, hosted the Blue Mind Men swim group or talked to me. Being part of the cold-water swimming community, starting at Tooting Bec Lido and now in the Lake District, he feels safe and able to express himself truthfully and openly. He's excited about the future now that he has found his niche and is surrounded by like-minded people: not just outdoor swimmers, but climbers, mountaineers, runners and photographers, all dedicated to their passion, but generous with their time and support.

'I love it. Some people do it for a specific mental health reason, but for me, jumping in as a fully acclimatised person is childlike, fun and makes me feel good. When I started, everyone said it's amazing, but there was no cited research. What we thought we knew is now being proven by science. For me, it's not at all about being macho or fighting the cold, or even controlled breathwork, like Wim Hof. It's more about relaxing into it and enjoying the feel of the cold on your body and what it's doing to your mind. I get my natural high.'

Oh Jonny, you are a die-hard raver!

TARA

Tara credits her husband for enticing her into the water about five years ago when he wanted some midlife adventure and told her he was going to investigate the local swimming club at Farleigh Hungerford, Somerset.[11] He said to her, 'You have to come with me in case I die.'

It annoyed her so much to see him enjoying himself in the water that she got in too and they began to swim together once a week. During lockdown she listened to a lot of podcasts and one in particular struck a chord. It was a life-coaching podcast and the life coach lived a few doors away from her. The coincidence needed to be explored, decided Tara, and she signed up for some sessions. 'I've always wanted to find my "thing" and, suddenly – wham! – I took a diploma and got qualified as a life coach. Of all the jobs I've ever had, this is the one where I feel most like me. My life looks similar, but inside I feel so different. If I can help anyone to change and have that same feeling, how amazing, what a privilege.'

We had two bars of 4G and hundreds of miles between us, but somehow our passion for cold water united us for a few brief seconds, enough time to share that special moment when you breathe in as your boobs meet the cold, and then lower your shoulders and breathe out slowly. Tara and I had been planning for me to drive down to where she lives, park Gloria up outside her house and find some cold water to swim in together while

11 The Farleigh & District Swimming Club, founded in 1933, is believed to be the oldest river-swimming club in the UK. It is sometimes referred to as the original 'wild swimming club'. Membership costs £12 per year, whether you swim just in the summer or all year round. Oddly, access to the field car park is only open in the summer months, so at any other time of year you have to park elsewhere and climb over the gate. Currently there are just over 5,000 members, mostly summer-only swimmers.

I interviewed her. But the evening before setting off, I just did not have the capacity to make the journey, which would have taken me down the M5 and flooded me with memories of going to visit my mum when she was still well and alive. Grief is a lonely place, but one I have to become familiar with until it feels more comfortable and I can look beyond its iron bars again. I phoned Tara to explain that I wasn't coming down, but could we work out an alternative way of being together in the water? I wanted to see where she swam and find out for myself why she loved it so much. So we arranged to meet on WhatsApp video the following morning and walk into the water together: her at Farleigh Hungerford and me at Crummock Water. Even though we were limited to a fuzzy picture, punctuated with broken sentences and squeals, it was easy to imagine how the other person was feeling because some things about cold-water swimming don't change: the initial shock, the cascade of emotions and then the transformation into calm.

As the geese joined us, I felt very relaxed, although irritated by the poor internet connection. So much of our lives has been lived through such communication over the last eighteen months: it's time it stopped. Nothing can replace actual physical encounters. But, on this occasion, it served a purpose, and saved petrol and wear and tear on Gloria and myself. It enabled us to embrace the cold water at the exact same moment and then disconnect while we each enjoyed our own solitary swims, ready to reconvene a few hours later back in our respective homes.

One of the most beautiful feelings I experienced that morning was a natural bond with a stranger, a few seconds of not feeling so alone in a place where I often find my rural isolation stifles me like a heavy cloak. Lightness and laughter competed with the honking geese, which seemed determined to outfox me, until I had the last laugh: just as I turned away and bent down to splish and splash at the water's edge, I heard them beat their wings into the deep lake and fly over my head towards the grassy area behind the beach. I caught them on camera because my phone was still videoing after my conversation with Tara.

Like me, Tara often gets home from swimming feeling energised, surfing on a wave of energy, so she quickly does housework and jobs because she knows she will feel tired and then hit a sudden wall. This morning her river was about 5.5 °C and the air temperature similar: a good balance, which felt comfortable both in and out of the water, with no wind chill to battle against.

Settling into our respective sofas, we started to chat. I really wanted to know whether Tara's change of direction career-wise had anything to do with cold-water swimming. There's nothing like putting your interviewee on the spot!

'I love connecting. Even as a child, I preferred to have one friend at a time. I love to be with one person at a time. I don't enjoy parties and small talk. Don't get me wrong,' Tara chuckled, 'I've got quite a few friends, but often see them separately and have a lovely time. And I've always been a doer, not a thinker. But after about three years of cold-water swimming I started to do more thinking. It was as if a part of my brain woke up after years of chasing around after other people, including many small children, as I was a teacher.

'I found space in the river particularly once I started going on my own,' said Tara. She had never done anything on her own before: she'd never lived on her own, had her children shortly after leaving university, always looked after her family and then started swimming, but with her husband, so it was a massive thing the first time she actually drove to the river on her own, got undressed, got into the water and swam alone. 'Life-changing' is how she described those first swims. It made her think about things more deeply: who she was, where she was in life and was she happy with life?

As we explored the connection between the cold water and its effect on our thought process, we both agreed that it could be transformational because when you turn your focus inwards, you see your raw state. No bullshit. Nowhere to hide, and the only person who knows when you're faking it is you.

'It's the thing that makes me feel most alive, and also there's a sense of bravery, invincibility and a profound stillness at the same time: a weird paradox. Sometimes I swim along the river, summer or winter, saying, "I am the river".'

Tara was serious. It was something even five years ago she would have dismissed as 'hippy stuff', but this connection to nature is now a huge part of swimming for her, especially in the river. And then she paused and thought again about what she'd just described.

'Actually, I mostly talk to myself when the water is warmer. I think I connect more with the outside in the summer, but in the winter, the cold drives me inside myself. My focal depth shrinks, my senses intensify as all thought, blood and emotion rush to my core. I notice the touch of the cold on my tummy, or my thigh or my ears, and concentrate on how it feels on just that tiny small piece of skin.'

I've not had much experience of swimming in rivers, only the Thames south of Oxford, and I must admit I found it quite terrifying because of the current. The tumbling, white water of our Lakeland becks is easier to engage with somehow: there is almost always an eddy to sit in, or a waterfall ready to give you a power shower.

'It's my river,' said Tara, and then asked whether that sounded mean or possessive. 'I don't mean I own it and don't want anyone else to swim there, but it's where I get a really deep feeling of space and a place where I feel comfortable because I've got to know it in detail. I don't really stay still in the river when it's cold.'

I remembered our video conversation and how she got into the river slowly and was still for a few seconds while we shared the moment and then she was off. She *always* moves and swims in the river.

'In winter I can only swim so far. So I set myself a landmark limit. I've swum there so many times I know the distances, and no matter how great I feel I won't go further than "that" tree. But if the kingfisher decides to fly past, I'd be frozen up watching it!'

I was reminded of the 'farting kingfisher' that taunts the Derwent river swooshers near Matlock by appearing when they least expect it and darting past their heads in a flash of blue. The vagaries of someone's keyboard had automatically changed 'darting' to 'farting' and the poor bird had remained windy ever since!

'I love the river and accept the different seasons and temperatures. By sticking strictly to swimming certain distances in winter, I know that I'm not going to see what's happening around the bend in the river for a good five to six months. The joy of the day when I think it's safe enough and warm enough to swim around the corner! I think to myself, I haven't been here since October. How exciting! I'll be able to swim up to Dingly Dell, Four Oaks, the campsites, etc. These landmarks mark the seasons and I'm going to get all those things back again as it warms up.'

Tara grew up in India, which she was always told probably gave her 'thin blood', and for most of her adult life she had to be somewhere hot: hot destinations for holidays, hot seas. People who've known her for a long time are slightly astounded by her love affair with the cold water. They say things like, 'This is quite weird, Tara ... I don't understand what's happened to you!'

'And I was never a sporty person or had a great relationship with my body. I used to think if someone had stuck me out in the wilderness I'd be dead within a minute. But, and I know this sounds a bit like "pride before a fall", but not many people do what I do: it's hard, it's uncomfortable and it carries risk. But now I can assess situations on a different level. I can do hard things, this cold thing, and survive and feel amazing. If someone left me in a cold place, I reckon I could last for ... half an hour!'

If someone left me in a cold place, I wonder how long I'd last. I think it would depend where I was, what was around me, how far away from help I was, how deep the water was – so many factors, so many ways of coping with the experience. But I know my adaptation to the cold per se has been informed by my cold-water swimming journey and, like so many of the people I've been talking with recently to write this book, it's been life-changing on many levels. I feel more ready than ever to be left in a cold place on my own and see how I cope.

But first, I want to share Tara's secret fantasy with you. It's one many cold-water swimmers have, but few of us make it a reality.

'I used to fantasise about having a lake at the bottom of our garden,' she confessed. Then she took me on her phone on a tour of her garden. After a few seconds she zoomed in on an ornate enamel bathtub. 'I had to shrink this fantasy down. Okay, so it's a bathtub, but it gets ice, thick enough to hack open with an axe. And I can sit in it any time I want and watch my toes turn blue. Here, I am forced to be still. But I don't do it daily. I hate daily practices. It feels too much like authority, something I'm not good with.

Why would I want to start telling myself I must do something?'

It's almost as if Tara wants to rediscover her inner child, rail against authority and play out late because she can.

'It's not an addiction, no, nothing like that. I don't need it, but I am having fun with it. I was horribly perimenopausal when I started swimming in the river: not unhappy, but beige, dismissive of everything, no real joy, just routine and acceptance. That first shock of the cold and subsequent elation reminded me about fun. And I haven't stopped wanting to have fun since. I can honestly say that cold-water swimming in my river has brought the "oomph" back into my life in so many ways.'

I love Tara's open curiosity about the cold, but in the same breath am surprised that she's not drawn to explore the frozen landscapes of Scandinavia or North America. 'It really scares me,' she admitted. 'I wouldn't do it off my own bat. If I knew someone in Scandinavia really well, and they said, "Come and stay, come and climb in my ice hole", I would probably do it, although I'd be bricking it. Is that the natural end of a cold-water swimmer's journey? Am I a real cold-water swimmer if I don't yearn to hang off a skimpy ladder and sink down into the dark water?'

ALICE

I think I might have got the job at Seasalt because during my job interview with Alice we talked about wild swimming! Although I didn't work there for long, it was the start of a friendship in and out of the water. Originally from Leeds, she moved up to the Lake District about six years ago. She has been swimming in Derwentwater near Keswick for around four years, first in a wetsuit, then for the last three years just a swimsuit. Not much will put Alice off swimming apart from particularly windy and wavy weather.

Can wind-up frogs also be control freaks? If so, then I'm sure Alice won't object to me attaching this description to her. If she does, I will be sure to hear about it!

The cold doesn't scare Alice – she may whinge about it as she's walking in, but admits that it's probably just noise for the sake of noise. If she wanted to walk straight back out, she would. She knows that as she walks in, her body is under control, putting one foot in front of the other, being careful not to trip over rocks, waiting a moment if she needs to and then stepping forward again. She is outwardly calm, but inwardly her brain is buzzing and fizzing almost out of control and then it slows down and comes to a stop – hence the wind-up toy analogy.

'I am a chronic overthinker, so the thing with the cold is from the moment you get in, and even if it doesn't last for the whole swim, it means I have to stop thinking about other things for a minute, five minutes, whatever it is; you have to stop concentrating on other things, because you are forcing your brain to concentrate on the moment.' It sounds as if the cold makes her brain just go, 'okay, we're here rather than anywhere else', and it stops thinking.

That release, even if just brief, is what Alice craves and why she loves the cold water. It feels to her as if her brain never switches off; getting to sleep can be an issue because she is always worrying about other people, something that's going on at work, or just nebulous other worries. As a self-confessed overthinker, she knows it is rare to have something that shuts her brain off.

Any thoughts she has as she's walking into the water are more connected to the feeling of that moment, like an automatic reaction to the particular body of water she's in. Every time we swim in Crummock Water, I'll hear her crooning about how clear the water is and how beautiful everything looks. Those are her Crummock lyrics; in Derwentwater she may sing a different song. However bad or good the day's been, there are always things in each place you swim that draw your focus, and it is specifically the cold that facilitates those feelings.

She's never afraid of how cold it might be because she is doing something she loves and knows she will feel that moment of release or escape within minutes of being in the water.

Given that her specific motivation for cold-water swimming is something so brief that it could possibly elude her, had she ever wondered whether she could try to prolong the feeling of release and escape? Her answer is an emphatic no. 'I know it's not going to last, and if I tried to make it last I'd lose it because I'd be thinking about how I can make it last longer. Also, I actually enjoy the different stages of a swim or dip. First the focus, no scatterbrained thinking here, the cold is making me focus on one thing and then I've transitioned into swimming, laughing, talking and I'm back. On reflection that's what it's like, but I've never thought of it as a process until you asked me!'

As an overthinker, Alice is prone to working issues out before taking action, but rarely if ever uses swimming as a time to reflect and troubleshoot. She usually swims with other people, but on the rare occasion she has swum solo finds it more difficult to concentrate on a complex problem because she's too aware of being on her own and needing to keep herself safe. On one occasion she swam alone out to the buoy in Bassenthwaite, which was fine to start with while her brain was switched off, but with no one to chatter with, her mind started to imagine there was something in the water with her. Not a good situation to be in, and now if she swims solo, she'll always swim along the shore rather than out into the middle of the lake so if she gets that same panicky feeling she can either stand up if it's shallow enough or swim closer to the edge and stand up.

'If I want to think things through, I go for a walk, but I always have something in my ears, either music or a podcast. Music gives me the perfect opportunity to zone out of what's around me and I allow the rhythm of the walking to help my brain think things through and I come to a solution by the end of the walk.'

For an aquatic creature who loves spending time in the water, Alice is strangely averse to getting her head wet or being underwater. When others are larking about in waterfall pools and trying to stick their heads behind the waterfall and peer through it, Alice always hangs back, watching but not joining in. And this is the paradox I see in a lot of swimmers: one small incident in childhood can knock their confidence for doing a particular thing in the water, but it doesn't stop them being in the water at every opportunity. Getting her face and head wet is nothing to do with the fear of her mascara running, but is directly related to an incident in the sea when she was about four years old. She was in a little rubber dinghy with a friend and a wave knocked it sideways, pitching them out so that she was momentarily trapped under the boat.

'I've never forgotten that, I can see it and feel it even now and I know I don't want to put myself in a situation where I would feel like that again. I have no need to do that to myself. I love watching other people jumping in off the jetty or doing a handstand in the lake, but I'm not going to do it myself. The only time I think about my near drowning is when it's wavy in the lake and then I can feel myself getting uncomfortable.'

Is it because you are afraid of not being in control? My question lands with a thud; I've hit the nail on the head. Not only is Alice an overthinker, but she is a control freak – both qualities readily acknowledged by her and likely to explain why she is how she is. Questions race through her mind in any given situation, such as, what if I can't control this situation? If I can't control it, what's the point of doing it? I know it's deep enough to jump off the jetty because I've just watched my friends jump off, but what if it isn't?

'On the jetty my brain is active and running through the ifs and buts like a pack of flash cards. But the moment I get in the water the questioning stops.' If I could get Alice in the water and on to the jetty in that order, I wonder if she would jump. I immediately suggest we go to Ashness Jetty while the lake is so high and the beautiful wooden structure that the launch calls in at on its way round Derwentwater will be knee-deep in water, even at the very end. Alice likes how I am thinking out of the box, but NO!

Talking of boxes, I ask her whether she has ever tried scuba diving. Absolutely not. The idea of it appeals, but would she want to do it? What if she ran out of air? What if she panicked? All reasonable questions and ones she knew she didn't have to ask herself because she knew she wasn't going to try it because she didn't want to be trapped in a box in deep water.

I know Alice is a brave woman, though, and I know she is tough. How else has she survived in retail for so many years? Her approach to managing staff at a retail outlet is similar to every other aspect in her life, apart from swimming. Control and overthinking. Working through processes and issues until everything is running smoothly and efficiently. If she can answer all her what-ifs, she is happy. So what is it about swimming that allows her to behave differently? To, dare I say it, let go, lose a tiny bit of control?

We go back to how she started swimming outdoors. Her friend Abby had said one day, 'Let's go swimming.' Alice had said no. Abby kept on suggesting it until Alice said yes. The first time they went they wore wetsuits and took a bottle of wine and two plastic cups for afterwards. It had been one of those revelation moments: an 'oh no, this is a whole new ballgame' moment. From being trussed up in a cheap wetsuit to swimming skins took no more than a few months and it is now highly unlikely that Alice will wear a wetsuit ever again.

'I feel more in tune with whatever water I'm in and in touch with my body. It feels more right. I like the physicality of it, rather than the slow anticipation of the water seeping into your wetsuit. I know I'm more vulnerable in just a swimsuit, but not in a bad way. Because I'm feeling everything I'm supposed to be feeling, I'm wanting to know what it's like to push myself further, to see what that feels like. If I think, no, I can't because it's cold, then I do it anyway. For me, there is nothing else that pushes you to that point of not wanting to turn back. Running you can stop, cycling get off and push, walking find another route, but swimming, of course you can turn back or not go in, but for some reason, especially if it's cold, I don't want to, I don't feel I can because I don't want to miss out on that moment I know I'll reach when everything feels amazing. It's almost a guaranteed pay-off.'

This sounds like she takes massive risks, but it's not about that at all. It can't be, because I know she has cancelled on occasion when it's been very windy or wavy. Many swimmers would do the same, but for Alice the cancelling isn't about being afraid of the rough water, but more about the fear of getting out into the lake and finding she's not enjoying it. She doesn't want to know how that sort of disappointment feels because she places such importance on what a swim means to her: a moment of peace that she can't get anywhere else.

Saying no to herself comes fairly easily, but it is only fairly recently that Alice has found the confidence to say no in a professional capacity, and she puts this down almost entirely to cold-water swimming. Her resilience to being uncomfortable in the cold has gradually built up over the last three years along with an increasingly more positive attitude to her body, not only what it can do, but how it looks. If she had asked herself even only a few years ago, before she moved up to the Lake District, whether she'd be stripping off down to a swimsuit with a bunch of other people on the side of a popular lake, she would have died laughing. No way would she have flashed flesh in public, let alone trotted off down to the water's edge and posed for a group selfie.

'Even when I'm not feeling great about myself, I still swim and get in a swimsuit alongside other people. I definitely wouldn't have done that in the recent past; I would have actively avoided that situation. It's because there's no judgement. That is a massive part of it. We all want to do it because we love it, not because we want to be slimmer, more daring, faster or wear sexier swimsuits than anyone else. Any competitiveness is playful between people who have got to know and trust each other well. If you can find a competitive bone in my body you can have my new Batoko swimsuit,' Alice laughs. 'You can win, you can have it, I'm not bothered.'

It's okay, I've got the Orca one, so we don't have a deal, Alice!

One of Alice's favourite swims was an ice swim one afternoon in Derwentwater. It was a beautiful day and they could see the ice further out towards the island, so they headed for that, excited to see how thick it was. Rather than being disappointed that it was only thin, they relished the crackling of the ice as they swam back and forth through it. She can't remember what she thought; her brain had completely relaxed after a difficult day at work and her body had just taken over and played with all the senses. It was the best feeling and the closest she thinks she's come to letting her inner child run free.

'But I'm not sure I have an inner child,' she says.

I don't want Alice to think there is anything wrong with not being in touch with that part of herself very often – overthinkers rarely are – but I've seen her floating across the Isthmus near Keswick on an inflatable pine-apple at least once and when I remind her of that afternoon, she tells me how as a child she had always wanted to be in the water wherever they were. At the seaside she would be the child who was just standing in the water up to her waist, not swimming, just standing. She remembers how the feel of the water around her had held her and allowed her imagination to roam free. The stories she made up and told herself while she was standing there were legendary in her family.

I think I am beginning to understand the real Alice, the one we have reached when we peel back the layers of self-control and constant what-ifs. Piecing together moments of creative imagination, great daring to even get in the water after her rubber dinghy experience, ensuring employees and friends feel cared for and inviting playful enjoyment with shards of ice, I have a near enough complete portrait of all of my five characters rolled up tightly in one person. Alice shows the qualities of the Mother, the Warrior, the Panther, the Child and the Thinker in everything she does. I feel she is on the brink of releasing the first four, but only if the Thinker in her is silenced.

What better place to silence the Thinker than to place it in an ice hole? One where risk is limited, so negative thought processes won't be triggered and we can allow the cold to do its job quickly and efficiently. It sounds as if I want to murder the Thinker in Alice!

And so I ask her whether she would be up for sitting in an ice hole. Is there anything that would make her not want to do it? If it was in a river with a flow and the danger of being swept under the ice and not being found until spring, then no, she wouldn't do it. It does happen, but I wasn't going to suggest that kind of ice hole!

'I'd definitely climb down a ladder, fixed or not, into an ice hole, yes. That doesn't scare me, the cold doesn't scare me, or slipping into the black water. I know I'd feel a bit of apprehension at the thought, but when the moment came, I'd do it.'

And what would give you that motivation? How do you know you'd do it?

'The cold. The absolute shock to the system. I want to feel that. I want to see what that feels like. To have that absolute silence in my head, bliss.'

THE ICE HOLE

At the beginning of this journey into the cold, I dreamt of my perfect ice hole. I imagined it would give me the answer to everything and I had a very clear image in mind: me, a hole in a frozen lake and the sun setting behind me.

I did get to sit in an ice hole. Three, actually. All three were completely different from each other and far from my perfect image.

The first was what I would call a 'proper' ice hole: a dark, roughly oval shape of water in a frozen fjord. I wasn't involved in making the hole and in a way that was disappointing, because that was the part I wanted to watch and understand.

On one of my trips to southern Norway at the end of 2021 I was lucky enough to do a spontaneous ice dip with a friend. We were on our way back from Kristiansand, the sun was going down and we were going to be driving straight past Elli's jetty. We knew there was quite a lot of ice on the fjord there, but had no idea whether it was still thick enough around the ladder or, conversely, whether it had iced over and we wouldn't have the right tools to break it open again. Our only tool was a fairly large axe, which looks great in a photo, but isn't very effective on real ice. Worth taking a look, though, because what else do you do on New Year's Eve while you're waiting to squeal at the hundreds of fireworks Norwegians love to let off at midnight?

The last time I had been on this jetty was on a windy night in early December, when I was staying with Elli to interview her for this book. The 'walk of death' had been terrifying that night, so I wasn't surprised to feel my stomach churning now as we walked down through the trees to the edge of the fjord. I was scared that the rocks and narrow planks of wood leading to the jetty would be iced over and lethal to walk on, but it seemed the stars were aligned and I began to relax and relish the time we had before it was too dark and too cold to be messing about in frozen water.

Everything was white except for the jetty itself, which just had a fragile coating of frost so you could see our footprints. The opaqueness of the ice indicated that it was still good and thick, but it was easy enough for my friend to bash away at the foot of the ladder to reopen the hole. While he was doing that, I gazed across the fjord to a few cabins, each draped in white twinkles as is now Norwegian tradition during the long, dark winter months. Once the hole was big enough for the two of us to bathe together, my friend stepped down on to the frozen fjord and walked out on to the ice.

My heart nearly leapt out of my chest, all my childhood fears of falling through ice whooshed into my head and I waited to hear a crack and a cry of help. But none came because the ice was at least a foot thick. I wish now that I had faced my fears and walked out myself. He placed the phone on its tripod on the ice, pointing towards the ever more beautiful sunset. Our window of opportunity was limited, though, so we had to stop faffing and get ourselves ready. I stripped off down to my bikini, pulled on my neoprene booties and gloves and picked up the hand-knitted Norwegian hat that Solveig had given me when I stayed with her.

With some upbeat music blasting out and creating Friday night party vibes, I felt the fire in my belly rising up. I wanted this so badly and nothing was going to stop me from doing it. Holding on to the steel ladder, I went down, one careful step at a time, my eyes focused on where I was placing my feet and not on the black water I was about to climb into. The fear had hold of me now, right at the base of my neck. My breath was slow and steady, in a conscious attempt to calm my nerves and prepare my body for the shock of the cold.

I used the memory of being here with Elli on that stormy night to motivate me: nothing could be as scary as that! I knew the water was deep here, maybe twenty feet, so the irrational part of my brain kept trying to signal danger, whispering things like 'What is going to be in the water with you?' I responded, 'Only what was here when I swam here before.'

I'd completely forgotten about the cold; it was almost irrelevant. Almost. Yes, it felt shocking as it crawled up my calves above my booties and then I felt its icy grasp as I lowered my bottom, keeping my feet firmly on the final rung, which was about two feet below the surface of the water. I was stuck in a semi-squatting position, my mouth hanging open and my breathing now out of control. I knew this was the moment of truth: I either lowered myself right down and let my feet dangle or I would have to climb back up the ladder. The thought that something was in the water watching my bum lowering, ready to eat it, was almost overpowering and I had to talk myself into being calm.

A few loud swears and pleas to my friend about how scary it was helped to shoo away the terrors, partly because he just grinned and agreed, but mostly because hearing my own voice meant I must still be alive!

I called on my Warrior as I let my feet slip off the bottom rung of the ladder. Deep breaths. The next step was to let go of the ladder and hold on to the edge of the hole, the ice itself. But that was slippery and went against all rational behaviour. 'Why would I deliberately hold on to something so insecure?' screamed my Thinker. The risk of my hands losing grip and my whole body being sucked down into the dark deepness below and vanishing under the miles of frozen fjord made common sense scream at me to climb back up the ladder.

If I wanted to do this, I had to get on with it. Every second spent assuming the worst would bring the worst closer to reality as I was gradually freezing to death (potentially, anyway!). Let your legs dangle! I had no choice if I wanted to move away from the ladder and use my arms to support me on the edge of the ice.

Vulnerability and exposure: two of the worst places to be mentally and emotionally, but I had to deliberately climb into them if I wanted to give myself this chance of a lifetime. If someone pulled the ladder away, would I ever be able to get out of this hole? Or would I need to wait and hope that the air temperature would miraculously warm up, the ice melt and I would swim to shore and scramble out, crying and whimpering?

Stop those thoughts. Don't think. Just do.

Do this, Sara.

My Warrior stood beside me and held me. You can do this. Slowly, I backed out into the circle of water and put my gloved hands on to the ice either side of me – it was strong, it was there for me, not against me, not my enemy, but my guardian. Allowing my entire being to cross that boundary of fear placed me in a different space where I wanted to stay and explore how it made me feel. In the ebb and flow of seconds passing, I remembered where I was and what was or was not below me. I felt panic rising like bile, acrid and sickening, but I swallowed it down and forced myself to get back into the space where I knew I would grow and flourish.

I turned around in the hole and placed my arms in front of me, crossed over on the ice, looking into the phone on its tripod across the ice from me. I think I smiled. I probably managed a grimace. The thing I wanted to do the most, but also wanted to do the least, was to feel under the ice, almost to see how thick it was, to brush its surface and know that it never saw the light because it always faced down into the dark depths. What would it look like if I was lying under it face upwards staring up at the world, separated by many inches of frozen water – would I see the face of my friend staring down in panic at me, or would I see nothing, like through thick gauze?

This was not a sensible line of thinking, as it made me wonder what it would feel like if something grabbed my ankle and the last thing I heard would be my friend calling my name – 'Saraaaaa!' – as I disappeared forever.

Then I remembered that he wanted to get in the ice hole too. So I watched as he climbed down the ladder one step at a time and joined me in our circle of frozen pleasure. My Panther decided it was exciting to have him in there with me and we kissed – ice kisses are the best because your lips are warm. Then we settled into our own feelings for a few seconds: a private space.

The sense of security his presence gave me made my Child want to play. I tipped forwards and let my legs float up behind me, my heels touching the undersurface of the ice; I reached down into the water and brushed the undersurface with my gloved hand – all the things I would not have dared to do on my own. My confidence was building and I felt totally comfortable in our ice hole.

It might sound weird, but I'd forgotten it was cold. Of course, I knew my body was in ice-cold water, but that information was somehow intangible, unlike the rough surface of the edge of ice against my bare arms. That was sharp and grazed me, but there was no pain because my arms were so cold. I wrapped my legs around my friend's waist and we kissed again, as if we were in tropical water, playful and carefree. When we swapped sides, both of us holding on to the ladder and him passing behind me, I could smell the warmth of his body close to mine and the contrast between cold ice and warm flesh was strangely erotic.

Our conversation seems random on the video, which I watched afterwards, and I can't remember what we talked about, but it was relaxed, content and irrelevant. We were both in our element: no fear, no anxiety, just peace. When it was time to get out, neither of us really felt the need or wanted to, but that must have been the danger zone creeping up on us.

But even once we had both climbed up the ladder, I knew I hadn't finished. I wanted to do a head dunk – there on my own in the ice hole. I took off my hat and my friend fussed about with placing it in the exact right place to look good in a photograph while I climbed back into the ice hole. I gripped the ladder and counted to three. That first dunk was incredible. I didn't notice the cold; I was too exhilarated. There was ice on my hair, and it whipped across my face as I surfaced: my eyes screwed tight shut and my mouth open in shock and pleasure. 'Whooooo,' I shouted – it felt absolutely bloody amazing. I wanted to go again. This time my friend brought my phone round and took the video from above me, shooting down to where the ladder dropped into the water. I bounced up and plunged down, the slushy black water closing over my head and my hair floating slightly on the surface. This time I broke free of the water with a cry of astonishment at how much colder this dunk felt than the first.

'You'd better get out now before you turn into an ice popsicle,' laughed my friend, who was itching to get back in and do a couple of dunks. I watched as he held on to the edge of the ice and dunked twice. Then we danced on the jetty like a pair of overexcited schoolkids, jiggling our now scarlet, swim-tanned bodies to stimulate rewarming through random muscle action.

I didn't want to get dressed, but I knew I should. Frozen bikini off and a thermal layer on. Foolishly, I'd left my extra layers in the truck because I had been worried that I would slip in the water as we teetered across the 'walk of death'! So all I had was my one thermal layer, no trousers, my Robie Robe swim cloak, a red hand-knitted hat and my socks and leather boots. The sun had set and the pinky-orangey skies wrapped around me instead, warming me from the outside in as I stood sipping piping-hot sugary gløg (non-alcoholic) as fast as I could. I knew it was the only way I might be able to stop the deep cold from consuming me completely. My entire body had tensed up and I ached like mad. I tried to consciously relax by bending my knees and doing mini squats and wiggling my hips around. Stiff muscles hurt and make it impossible to feel warm as cold blood streams back through your heart. I felt uncomfortable and like a statue. Was I already a popsicle? This was the coldest I'd been since my Black Moss Pot fiasco and, I realised, had the potential to be more severe than that. Thank goodness we'd called time when we did. As the blood recirculates back through your heart there is a further drop in core temperature and we were certainly close to 32 °C, mild hypothermia. I felt in touch with reality, I could make sense of where I was and what I was doing, but was starting to feel an almost overwhelming urge to lie down and go to sleep there on the jetty as darkness billowed down around us.

Every inch of me was in chaos: utter bliss and happiness and near panic survival mode. Time to get off the jetty and walk back up to the truck, put more layers of clothes on, sip more hot drink and crank up the heater while we were driving back home.

Forty-five minutes later, the cold had really set in and I was just not warming up as fast I do normally. While the sauna was heating up, I did some yoga stretches just to keep moving. It hurt to bend my legs and to move. My back ached low down, where my kidneys are, so I did lots of rubbing and stretching just to intensify the rate at which my circulation was working. Gradually, the pain was easing and by the time I was sitting in the sauna I felt warmish. It was 61 °C and intense. To cope with my slight nausea and light-headedness, we opened the door a crack now and again so I could find air. Normally, it takes around thirty minutes to start to sweat in this 'dry sauna', but within only around five minutes my skin was wet – the speed at which my body was now rewarming was incredible, but instead of being relieved, I just felt overwhelmed. The ice hole experience had been a holistic one: my body and mind had been exposed to extreme cold and extreme sensation. It would take a while to process what had happened.

I needed to get out of the heat and so I went to lie down in the cooler bedroom. It took half an hour before I felt the nausea and prickly heat leave my body and another ten minutes for my headache to start to dissipate. My friend brought me a glass of cold apple juice with ginger, put a wet, cold flannel across my brow and sat with me to make sure I was safe (men can be Mothers too). After an hour or so, with my thirst quenched, I was ready to think about celebrating New Year's Eve.

Later, in the calm after the fireworks from all sides of the fjord, I reflected on the afternoon and how it had affected me so deeply. My conclusion is a flash of inspiration, not carefully thought through. But it really felt as if the real magic hadn't been down to the coldness of the water or ice, but the rarity, the gift, the chance of a lifetime, to be in such a cruel and harsh place and survive, to be truly living. An extreme slice of opportunity where time, circumstance and nature all align.

The second ice hole I sat in was quite a different experience and taught me so much about the uncertainty of ice holes. They are not all beautiful or aesthetically pleasing and the sun does not always set behind you, giving you a rosy glow. Circumstances, technical hiccups and time constraints can all work against you. But that is the reality of ice bathing.

It is perfectly possible to create your dream ice hole in the middle of a lake, but you need a chainsaw with a very long blade or an ice saw and plenty of experience! Most ice holes are actually found at the foot of a fixed ladder, or close to the edge of a lake where you can stand on the bottom of the hole and crouch down into a sitting position. When cutting the hole, it is far safer to cut a triangle shape, so that you can use the narrow end to get out of the hole more easily by placing your elbows on the surface of the ice as anchors. In a square or oblong hole with slippery sides but no ladder and no safe exit strategy, things could get tricky quickly. Popular in countries such as Sweden and Finland, a ready-made hole that is kept permanently open using some kind of warm air flow system, and preferably a wooden box fitted inside the hole and a lid, seems like a good option too.

Knowing that we weren't going to be cutting our hole out in the middle of the lake made me feel slightly more comfortable about following my friend across the frozen lake on a wet and windy night in early February. We had done a recce the previous afternoon while the sun was setting and if the chainsaw had been long enough we may well have created our perfect ice hole. However, the ice was far thicker than we expected, even only about twenty feet from the lakeshore, and the chainsaw we had was nowhere near long enough. It was the only tool we had available, so we had to abort the mission and think of an alternative plan (the Thinkers working together).

The following day we waited to hear from someone who had a much longer chainsaw, but he was using it in the forest. February is when Norwegians always cut wood for the following winter. It's just what you do. So we waited. The weather deteriorated and the thought of ice holes took on an ever more ominous hue. Why were we going to do this? Our final evening together and we were going to walk out on to a frozen lake in the rain and attempt to cut an ice hole fit for two, or would it just be for one? As the weather grew worse and night closed in on us, we set off inland some twenty miles or so to collect the chainsaw and get cracking.

Walking out for the second time to the same place on the ice felt marginally less terrifying because I'd done it before and survived, but being left alone on the ice with just the ambient night sky surrounding me while my friend trudged back to his truck to fetch the axe pushed me to my limit. I could see the halogen light he carried disappearing from the lake and into the trees. There wasn't a sound except for the pitter-patter of rain on the surface of the ice and an eerie whistle as a gust of wind whipped through the tall trees on the lakeshore. I stood on about eighteen inches of ice and beneath me I had no idea how deep the water was. It wasn't far to the safety of solid ground, but I was rooted to the spot. All I dared to do was tread around in roughly the same area, keeping an eye out all around for anything that might be creeping up on me. My imagination was having a riot! This solitary wait only lasted about ten minutes, but it felt like I had been abandoned to the wolves. Then my heart leapt as I saw the light twinkling in the trees and I knew he was coming back for me.

The sound of the chainsaw firing up did something to my insides, but not in a good way. Some women find burly lumberjacks sexy, but, although I am usually one of those ladies, that night I just felt absolutely terrified. No logs for a cosy fire. No snuggling up together in front of said cosy fire. No. It felt as if we were only out there because of some mad desire of mine to experience the whole process of making and sitting in my very own ice hole.

With the main triangle now cut, the task of lifting out the ice proved tricky without ice tongs and caused lots of huffing, puffing and swearing. I was standing a safe distance away, holding the light, and could see that this ice was not playing fair with us. My friend chopped it up with the chainsaw into smaller chunks and tried to push each one down into the water and slide it under another chunk. The plan was a bit like 'Squares', where you create a space and then can move all the other pieces more easily. But the first chunk kept bobbing back up.

I could feel my jaw tensing every time a chunk was pushed down, praying it would stay down and the one next to it could be released. The rain was getting heavier and the risk of the battery on the light running out was growing higher. At last, the first piece was out. Every last ice chunk had to be manhandled out of the hole and pushed across the ice, where we stood it on its end to create a sculpture. The uneasy feeling in my guts grew stronger. However, after all this effort, I had no option but to get in the hole.

'How deep is it?' My voice sounded like a small child's, almost a whimper. My friend poked the stick he had been trying to use to heave out the ice blocks down into the water as a measuring tool. It only sank into the water about two feet. My relief was almost audible! Suddenly it seemed doable, and in spite of the rain, wind and darkness I began to get excited. The only deterrent was the colour of the water. It wasn't black and forbidding, but murky and muddy-looking. God knows what was on the bottom of the lake, but I was about to find out! I would either be able to stand and then crouch down, or I would sink in and have to be pulled out.

Once my friend was satisfied with the hole and how he had arranged the ice sculptures around one end of it, he set up the phone on its tripod and we were ready. The feeling rippling through my body was amazing. I felt on fire and physically aroused. The surface of the ice around the lake seemed solid, although it had melted slightly where we had been standing. Perversely, I loved the feeling of rain on my skin, wetting me through ready for full immersion. It was almost like foreplay before the main event!

We had no music, just the pitter-patter of sleety rain on ice and my purposeful breath as I slipped down into the water, with my arms crooked and my hands holding on to each side of the hole. I watched as my thighs submerged and then my feet met something squidgy and I sank up to my ankles. I groaned and hoped there was solid ground down there some-where and not just stinky rotten vegetation, or worse! It reminded me of the times I have stepped into one of those tiny mountain tarns that you just happen to come across on a walk and as your foot goes through a sort of crust under the water into potentially bottomless softness, you pray it's not the decomposing body of a long-lost hiker. Grim, but that's how my mind works.

Once settled into the murkiness, I relaxed and allowed the stillness of the night to hug me. I didn't know if this was the last time I would sit in an ice hole, I didn't know whether I would get the opportunity to have another go and make a more beautiful one, but it was my ice hole. My companion didn't want to sit in it – the debatable bottom made his skin crawl; whereas for me, having my feet on some sort of ground gave me the confidence to relax into it. Our fairy lights were wrapped around the ice sculptures, and far away on the opposite side of the frozen lake, faint orange lights from a cluster of houses reassured me. I felt this was pretty close to that imaginary perfect ice hole at sunset.

Reluctantly, I climbed back out, feeling powerful and empowered in my beautiful red bikini. Time to get dressed, pack up our few tools and walk back to the warmth and safety of the truck.

My final, and most important, ice hole was back on home turf.

It isn't very often that I have both my children together with me at home at the same time. Emily lives with her boyfriend in Sheffield; Robin has his own life too. The dynamics of our relationship have changed over the years and these days our roles within it are more interchangeable. I am not the sole carer any more; they care for me too. Tough love is the kind of love I have given them, not of free choice, but circumstance. Our conversations are wide-ranging, often edgy, and we know which buttons to push and not push.

Consequently, we don't often clash, but when we do it can be painful. Mostly, it is almost as if we need to re-establish a hierarchy when we get together again. Often, the first hours are blissful reconnection, the middle ones a mini battle of wills and in the final ones we're okay again and don't want to be apart. Is every deep relationship like this?

The plan was to walk up to Scales Tarn on my favourite mountain, Blencathra. I had a feeling the tarn might be partially frozen as we'd had a smattering of snow and a few low night-time temperatures. Getting three of us out of the house fully loaded with a picnic, enough layers (what I considered enough for the mountains in winter) and suitable footwear, and without forgetting something major, was a Herculean task, even now, as three adults. If I'd just stepped back and packed my own bag and then waited by the front door, or on the sofa, calmly, I'm sure it would all have been fine. Or at least, might have been, until we reached the foot of the track and someone realised they'd forgotten a coat.

I think that's the eternal curse of motherhood, always has been and probably always will be, no matter how old my offspring are. And why would anyone want to wear shorts in early February on a walk up a Lakeland mountain? My son agreed to take a pair of bottoms with him just in case. I wasn't bothered so much about him being cold per se, more about how cross I'd feel if he whinged and rushed what we were doing, especially up at the tarn. I knew how exposed and windswept it could be up there and we'd got previous experience of walks being curtailed for this very reason!

My expectation was to revel in their company in a place I adore. The reality slipped its halo on the way up the track. A heavy lump of sadness sat in my chest and I had no idea why. Memories of other walks I'd done up here? Mostly on my own and wishing someone else was with me.

Thoughts about all the years I'd lived in this area and how many times I'd walked up here ... and I just felt so bloody lonely and low.

I really needed to move away, start afresh.

I felt as if I was trudging up there like a hamster on a treadmill and not really connected to anything around me. Emily overheated and tried to pass me her coat. A small thing, but it triggered a massive reaction in me. All those years of being the one to carry her purse, her coat, herself, her phone ... always me, always me doing the looking after, the weight-bearing – who looked after me? Who carried my picnic in their rucksack and made sure I was okay on the footpath? I was crying. I was bloody crying out there on a public footpath in front of my two young adult children.

I stopped and looked back a couple of times and saw Robin getting nearer to me, carrying Emily's coat. Then I felt a tugging on my rucksack and I swung round. He was trying to attach it to the rucksack and get me to carry it anyway! And he was laughing, Emily was laughing.

Stop! I told myself. Look at yourself. Remember what you *are* capable of doing. Remember that if you can walk into cold water or sit in an ice hole in the dark, then you are brave enough to face life alone ... to live life alone.

As quickly and heavily as the mood cloud had sunk over me, once we crested the top of the footpath and were standing on the Common, a place of stunning views and paragliding, it dissipated. I breathed in the cold air and allowed the fog in my head to clear. Shame at having spoilt the beginning of our day made me pull Emily and Robin into a tight embrace. Now I felt better and ready to be in the moment.

With the clag hanging down over Sharp Edge I seriously doubted that Emily would be able to walk on up to the flat summit of Blencathra, but we agreed to reassess this once we had reached the tarn. I suspected there would be quite an icy path up the left-hand side of the tarn.

Scales Tarn lies in a corrie formed in the Ice Age; it's a dramatic setting, with Sharp Edge rising up to the right and the back wall of the tarn sliding down into the black water. As the path flattens off, you get your first view and I squealed in delight: 'Ice'. It was there. The tarn wasn't completely covered in thick, white ice, but was definitely frozen over in places, especially close to where we were going to sit and have our picnic. My little axe, strapped on to my rucksack, quivered in delight and I could hardly wait to strip off and get in and do some chopping.

I asked Emily if she would take some really good photos of me in the ice. A slow but bubbly feeling was rising up from my stomach. This was the place I wanted to be, these were the people I wanted to be with. I was excited to relax into the icy bath, and listened to the cautions of my children with half an ear. I wasn't scared or nervous; I just wanted to get in. We agreed that I'd only go in as far as my knees and then sit down. Emily perched on a rock that jutted out of the ice and watched me as I started to use the axe to make a little channel to walk through. Although the ice was paper-thin, it was sharp and sounded like glass as it tinkled and crackled from my axe tapping or from my gloved hands pushing down on it in front of my legs. I knew the water was cold, of course – there was a layer of ice – but it didn't feel cold. I was in my element and unaware of time passing. I knew what photo I wanted and I had to get to the spot where the water would be deep enough to sit down, but not too deep so as to worry the children. It was painful, slow work. But if I'd just marched through, which would have been difficult anyway because the rocks are always uneven and slippery here, my shins and calves would have been bleeding messes and caused even more alarm. Every time I pushed down with my hands, the broken ice slid up my forearms and grazed them – no blood drawn, but an itchy, uncomfortable feeling.

No walkers appeared at the top of the path, but there was a small group working their way up the rocky path to the beginning of Sharp Edge. We had the place to ourselves. I was in my own little world, but very aware of Emily and Robin watching me and telling me what to do and not do. It was as if they didn't understand that I knew what I was doing. I wasn't afraid, but they were. For me.

And then it hit me. I am cared about. I am valued. I am their mother and I mean the world to them. Instead of feeling like a huge responsibility, motherhood suddenly felt like a giant hug. They may not have understood what I was doing, or why I was doing it, that much they made clear in the way that they were telling me off for wanting to slide under the ice and for wanting Emily to take a photo of my legs through the ice, and in how appalled they were at the blood dripping down my right shin where the ice had cut me. Why had I ever doubted my role in their life, or in fact in the lives of other people who I value and love? This place, an ancient, all-consuming place of memories, was my place. This ice was the ice that I had been searching for and it had been here all the time.

Maybe it's only by travelling away from my core and reaching out to like-minded people who are connected to me by the water, the cold water, that I have been able to understand myself, find the missing piece to myself?

Maybe there is nothing missing? Am I complete, just a bit broken after too many punctures to my lungs?

As I hunkered down on to the rocky, but reassuringly firm, bottom of Scales Tarn with the cold water seeping up to my shoulders and the tinkling ice grazing my upper arms and knees, I looked at Emily and Robin – my beautiful children who would not be here if I wasn't. I smiled at Emily's phone, through to the digital world into which I had tried to escape.

I needed both: this safe space here with my own flesh and blood, and that world out there with my fellow cold-water selkies. In both places I now know my worth.

'You have everything you need.' The Dutch hypnotherapist had pre-empted the words of all the people I had met: the Mother, the Warrior, the Child, the Panther and the Thinker. They are all within me and within us all. We bring them out in each other and can bring them out in ourselves. The cold water is the window to our true selves, and by opening that window to others we become a community.

The cold water has taught me to love myself in a different way. The ache of uncertainty, a sense of aloneness and fear may still be there and probably always will be, but when I'm in the water I find brief moments of no tension, no holding back, no nothing, just me. That ache is temporarily filled.

The cold is an opportunity to open up completely, to empty my head of all negative thoughts, all thoughts. I feel on a cellular level and am completely in the moment, present and yet far away. The pain as my nerves resist the cold is a barrier that I enjoy stepping over, with intent and purpose. On the other side of the pain are freedom, clarity and lightness: the cold fix.

Yes, it's like being an addict in many ways, but it is a natural high and some days we need a bigger dose than others. But it is free ... the only price we pay is time.

I went in search of good cold water to see if it would help me find the parts of myself that went missing at some point in my life. I talked with a bunch of strangers who share my passion for cold water to see if they could help me unlock the key to the missing pieces. Together we worked through all our emotions, stories and reasons why we believe the cold water completes us. We may not fully understand how it happens, however many podcasts, social media posts and books written by experts and scientists we consume. All we know is that we need the cold fix.

I don't exactly know when I realised I was broken – I had assumed it was when the surgeon cracked open my bones to fix my legs because that is the point at which I lost my connection to my physical life. But it may have happened even before I was born. Are any of us born whole? Do we need life and others to complete us or to chalk doodles on the blank slate of our being?

When I was in Ryan's workshop and felt something leap out of my body and scuttle into the corner, I believe it was the Thinker in me, the one that was often negative and unable to face up to the truth for fear of being hurt or hurting others. I've learnt that in relationships, whether those are romantic or family or friends, we so often dance around the elephant in the room. The elephant might be disconnection, lies, betrayal, distance, hurt, pain, discomfort ... we don't want to face it and deal with it. So we bury our heads in illusions: ones that are more comfortable, ones of 'connection' and 'safety'. We decide not to talk about that 'thing' because it is just too difficult. But the truth doesn't just go away. I think it can live in a shadowy place, which might explain why I originally saw this 'Thinker' figure as scuttling around, with a frown and a degree of meanness about it. Our inner critic perhaps, the shadow-based coping mechanisms we adopt when we know we want to say something, but aren't brave enough to.

So, if that is the case, was I living a lie for a long time? Did I only start to live the truth when I went into a state of deep breathing in the workshop? Or would I have gone there anyway through my cold-water swimming?

One thing I believe is you will never learn to love yourself if you know you're hiding things from yourself and others.

But it takes time and there is definitely a 'right' time to come out of the shadows and bring the truth forward into the light and hold it up in its raw state. Our path through life can be so convoluted or traumatic that the only option we feel we have is to hold on to the truth for too long or, worse still, to never let others see it.

I'm just so relieved and grateful to have been given the opportunity to experience the power of the cold water. If I hadn't had that operation, if I hadn't lived in the Lake District with easy access to cold water, if my children hadn't been brave enough to come into the water with me while I was still on crutches, if I hadn't had the tenacity to push myself out of my comfort zone into ever colder water … there are so many scenarios and rabbit holes into which I could have disappeared. But I hope I now know how to use the tools that lie within me to become the person I want to be, with the Mother, the Warrior, the Child, the Panther and the Thinker I want to have by my side: kind, brave, inquisitive, bold and positive.

Someone asked me recently whether I would dig out my Club des Cinglés card and take on the Giant of Provence if I could have my cycling fitness and strength back again for just one day?

No, I said. I don't feel the need to prove myself any more. I am enough.

But it takes effort, commitment and self-care to find the balance between just being alive and living. All the people I interviewed are testament to searching for and striving to find this balance.

The cold is their friend, their lover, their teacher, and is often the only constant in their life. When the world is in flux, many have found peace and stability in the cold. It is a place where anxiety, grief, loss, confusion, pain and tiredness go to lie down with angels. And while you breathe, close your eyes, soften into the discomfort of the cold, these angels wash your being in silence and re-cloak you as you leave the water.

A beautiful combination of spiritual, science, emotional and physical, the cold water provides safety in the depths of risk, comfort in the arms of discomfort and pleasure amidst pain. We are not masochists; we are ordinary humans who have found a way to live while we're alive.

CONTRIBUTORS

CLAUDIA
@creationclaudia

SARAH
@adventure_sair

SOLVEIG
@solsidencoaching

ELLI
@lifeisnow_behappy

LEELOU
@lakes_dionaiad

JOHNNIE
@fruitionlab

RYAN
@urban_ice_tribe

FIEN
@feelslikefiente

ELAINE
@rebellelarousse

JAY
@covidicebath

MATTY
@iswim_and_iceswim

JONNY
@jonnyhcowie

JAIMIE
@jaimie.monahan

TARA
@wildswimmingwoman

RORY
@rorysouthworth

ALICE
@alice_mitch90

ACKNOWLEDGEMENTS

Writing a book about yourself is not an ego trip; it is a humbling experience, especially when you start to see yourself through the eyes of others. Those others include members of my family, notably my late father and mother, my daughter, Emily, and my son, Robin.

My father used to describe himself as a 'silverback', as in gorilla! He was referring to his excessively hairy chest, which went silver as he aged. He had a stroke aged fifty-six and spent the next twenty years living a restricted lifestyle, semi-paralysed and with dysphasia, which allowed him only limited speech. It was a cruel fate for such an active, capable and practical man, who was doing head dips on his windsurfer and handstands right up until the day before his stroke. I watched him suffer and retreat into himself away from a world he could no longer be a part of. I saw my mother devoting her life to care for him and this taught me the meaning of unconditional love.

When my mother took on the challenge of caring for me after my surgery, I felt enormously guilty for putting her in the position of carer again, especially during those difficult moments when we clashed over silly things. It took a while for us both to heal from those moments. But we did and we became close again. She always believed in my writing and we spent many hours discussing plots and characters for various books I started over the years. Sadly, neither of them lived to see my childhood dream of becoming a published author come true, but I know they know.

Emily and Robin found our roles were suddenly reversed, and whereas as their mother I had always been their rock, there have been many occasions over the last six years or so when I have been forced to lean on them for my daily needs and emotional reassurance. But we have always been a strong team and I know we always will be.

It was Robin and his girlfriend, Aimée, who listened to my ramblings and helped me draft the initial email/proposal to Vertebrate Publishing while we were driving to the Ardnamurchan Peninsula in Gloria, my VW campervan. A patient Emily listened to me reading out chunks of an early draft while she commuted to work and provided essential constructive criticism along with the idea of incorporating my 'family' of Warrior, Mother, Child, Panther and Thinker.

Kirsty Reade and the whole team at Vertebrate Publishing bore the brunt of my tweaks, questions and suggestions until a final draft of *The Cold Fix* emerged months later. Thank you for taking that leap of faith and welcoming me into the Vertebrate family.

But I know that I wouldn't have been able to create the multi-layered meat of this book without the love, support and integrity of the sixteen cold-water swimmers and dippers from around the world who gave up their time, invited me into their lives and homes and willingly shared their innermost experiences and hopes with me. Warriors, Mothers, Children, Panthers and Thinkers: we are all part of each other's stories now. Thank you: Ryan, Jaimie, Elaine and Matty; Claudia, Solveig and Leelou; Rory and Sarah; Fien, Johnnie and Elli; Jay, Jonny, Tara and Alice.

And, finally, thank you Readers. Whether or not you love the cold, or even swimming, I hope that you have found moments of joy, hope and tenderness in these pages, moments that you can carry with you on your own journeys so that together we can try to spread some good stuff in this crazy, noisy and ever-spinning world of ours.

Q & A

I ask the questions, other cold-water swimmers give the answers!

 How does your body react to cold water? Do you love a good shiver? Are you frankly terrified of shivering?

If I stay in even a little too long, I have about five minutes once I get out before I start shivering violently. So I prioritise getting dry and into warm clothes and hopefully managing a few sips of a hot drink before the shaking starts! I don't love the shivering as it creates overwhelming, extreme muscular tension throughout my body, especially in my jaw (causing rare moments of silence!) and back. It lasts maybe ten minutes and then I usually feel fine, though I have to admit to sometimes cuddling a hot water bottle and cranking up the heating for the drive home.

A hot water bottle makes me feel sick, so even if I got the shivers I couldn't bear to use one.

I used to say that I *love* the cold, but I hate *freezing* (I love a hot water bottle at night), but I seldom freeze and shiver after a swim in the cold sea. My go-to is a small bucket and a Thermos with boiling hot water. I pour it into the bucket before jumping in the sea, and it's perfect to put my feet in while I dry myself and get dressed. Often I get into the sea several times.

Skins, my shiver is decent. I'd say it's intermittent rather than constant, but definitely a lot of movement in it.

My shiver is more of a rumble.

I love to shiver and then dance.

I honestly do not mind a shiver sometimes … I do change outta wet stuff right away; some don't … I find wool garments work really well in warming naturally and moving my body … some good old-fashioned jumping jacks get things flowing again. Warm drink always; alcohol makes it worse! Heated seats in one's car are an added bonus for the ride home if there is a journey, but before I had them I used a hot water bottle. And ultimately, if you just can't get warm yourself, a shower, sauna or steam room, which I personally try to end with a cool shower before I walk out and dry off. I'm all for regulating naturally but not if you're feeling miserably cold. Defeats the purpose, I feel … there are many protocols on this, but I just do what works for me.

I shiver regularly … but can deal with it. I once tried a warm shower (not hot) but it was terrible! I had the impression I was burning from the inside – so not for me. I prefer walking very quickly, drink hot tea, of course, and warm up in front of the fireplace.

I've still not popped my shiver!

I dry off and get out of my costume immediately and put my bathrobe or PJs. I have a long thick padded coat too. Cup of coffee and biscuits, whilst my toes and feet catch up with warming up. Also, parts of my body still feel wet even when dressed, but it's the sensation of the cold exposure.

Shivering is a normal part of the after swim/dip for me. When I first
started OWS last year, my teeth would literally be chattering
uncontrollably and I was unable to hold my cup without spilling
anything. I still shiver now, but it's a lot less and I now try to relax into
it as well, rather than tensing up.

I don't tend to shiver, but it happened once when there was a really
strong cold wind and I took too long to get myself dried and wrapped
up, also had a long walk back up the bay that day as it was a very low
tide and I realised I had forgotten my dry shoes. It wasn't a pleasant
experience and took me a good few hours to warm up again.

I shiver when I'm tired and sat in a perfectly warm room, but so far I've
never shivered when cold-water dipping … my body and mind seem to
be more prepared for that somehow. Although I've 'fizzed' so much
that I wasn't sure if I could use my hands to dress myself.

Once it gets cold I always shiver. The descent into shivering starts
within five to ten minutes. The first time it happened was worrying.
I know I could avoid it by reducing the time in the water; however,
it is now part of the swim experience for me and I enjoy the process
of rewarming.

I shiver in the breeze after a long swim when the cold stealthily seeps
into my bones and I stagger out of the lake. I'm euphoric in the
drunken state, but grey clouds often hide the afternoon warmth and
I shake uncontrollably. Usually the wind whips up across Crummock
as I change, struggling to pull on layers. A usual daily swim in summer!
I have to concentrate to walk back to the car and have the
heater on full blast.

I tend to go numb while getting dressed, and then feel the coldness
to the bone for quite some time afterwards. But I understand what
you mean about the lack of clattering teeth.

I rarely shiver from the cold while cold-water swimming or dipping. Doing it for a few years now, I noticed I can warm my body from the inside out. I don't do the Russian method, with the warming up, and not always the Wim Hof breathwork method either. Cos I don't need the preparation any more. If I feel cold afterwards, which seldom happens, I drink ginger tea or go for a walk.

I do love a good shiver and expand it into a wiggle and a jiggle.

Nothing beats a hot tea after ice swimming.

New to cold-water swimming, four months in, I shake like crazy. I now fear the getting out as opposed to the getting in. Does this improve? I get dressed quickly, do the hot drink, hot water bottle and tons of layers, but not improved as yet. Dips are around twenty minutes, ten minutes if like 4 °C.

 Feel free to tell me what a cold-water bath/dip/plunge/swim brings to your life that nothing else can.

If I sit in my tub first thing in the morning after yoga I can literally feel my world change colour: always to a brighter, more intense shade or hue.

It gives me *me* time and powerful feelings for the whole day.

Samadhi for me! I am so grateful.

Fire! It fuels the fire of life in my belly!!

I've had the *worst* day, and all I could think of was getting submerged somewhere. And I did, and I came out a different, better me. Can't explain it. It just works.

Free from pain in my hand for some hours.
Newborn every 'down under'.

Dipping like you say always elevates one's mood. It's simply ridiculous.

Quietness in my head ... is that even a word? RESET. Those are the 'noisy squirrels' I talk about. It feels like freedom when they shut up for a moment or two!

A whole body tingly buzz which lasts for hours, happy, fizzy.

Full of giggles and understanding about commitment to self-care when doing cold-water exposure.

When my world is only shades of black and white, my daily dip gives me the perspective to finally see colours again!

It's an immense sense of freedom. Almost in a sensual way. I feel alive, strong, girly, playful, free, carried, weightless in the water. The cold is challenging. The waves break on my body. The full immersion hits my brain and gives me a kick in the arse. I go alone, and being trustful and brave enough to count on my own strength and knowledge, feeling my body and its limits, gives me sort of a proud and fulfilled feeling. I can do this! I can do anything! And it's passion, the kiss on my skin. The embrace of the water.

Your beautiful words are so true to my heart! Aren't we lucky to have found the secret reset button?

Because it's time I've set aside just for me and my cold-water experience, I find it very grounding. I reconnect with myself and my body. Just for those few moments, nothing else and no one else matters. And when I get out I'm cheerful and calm and better able to care about everything and everyone.

Does the cold water improve your body confidence?

Totally. To be fair, it was the wild swimming initially in warmer (well, not much, it is the UK) waters that helped with body confidence. Getting undressed and dressed on a river bank with lots of people around (usually fully dressed, overdressed walkers) escalates your sense of 'I just don't have time to give a F about this', and then when I first started cold-water dipping I felt so grateful for a body that can do hard things; it really changed my perspective. Now, instead of wishing my body away (I wish I had … I wish I didn't have …) I say thank you to my body for all the fun in life it lets me have. Oh, and another thing, after a sub-5° dip your fingers can't really hold up towels, etc., so you do flash a lot of passers-by. Ooops, sorry everyone in the south-west!

It is strange, yes, to think I once hated parts of my body but now accept they're mine and therefore special.

True! And just enjoying the sensations of the cold replaces many negative self-criticisms.

Strangely enough, now that you ask, and I therefore think about it … yes, I don't hate my body any more!

I'm still wild swimming in shorts. I don't have massive body issues … self-criticism is high, though, regarding my thighs. The cold water makes me forget all that, though. When you are in ice-cold water, there is only room for one thought!

The strength I see in my body doing this has made me confident. I realise I'm capable of so much in all areas of life. I felt nervous at the gym this year learning to train with weights. Then it hit me: you do something likely no one else here does. You're strong. You can do this too.

I can say that it has definitely increased my confidence around my naked body. I would've never shared some of the things I have without the cold water. Love you, Sara. You're always an inspiration.

Body confidence 100% threw away all my mind-chattering about how I look in a swimsuit since I started the journey of cold-water exposure. Wearing a swimsuit or a bikini is part of the fun, knocking down any negativity of what I look like or what others may say. Pre water immersion, I would never contemplate exposing my body. Now, after a year, I feel my confidence has grown to not care about image as long as I have put on my lipstick.

For me, at fifty-eight, feeling 'sexy' is something swimming has helped me rediscover after some years of not understanding the concept or not allowing myself or not being 'allowed' by the people I had in my life to believe I could be. Now, I feel at my 'sexiest' when I'm doing or have done something extraordinary. The fire I feel roaring inside me is tangible. All others see is a glow. It's nothing to do with make-up for me, but how high the flames are inside. If I picked through the frames of my GoPro videos one by one, I'd cringe at body bits I think look horrid, ugh. It's not about those bits, though, is it?

I know what you mean about scrolling through the images and feeling a bit ugh. I don't think I ever look in the mirror and think, yeah, I'm sexy – and that's been true at all sizes, shapes and ages of me, even when I was a slimmer gym bunny, dressed up for a night out. For me, I think I feel it in the interactions with others – when you have a connection with someone, when you 'get' each other, when you make each other laugh, when there's a moment of emotional intimacy, and yes, in those moments when we feel capable, strong and confident in our body's ability, regardless of shape. I don't know if that's quite a female interpretation of feeling sexy – I imagine men interpret it in a much more physical/aesthetic way. Wild swimming definitely helps with both of those – the feeling capable and those moments of connection, which feel even more so through adversity (winter swimming and river swimming can feel quite adverse at times!).

I agree that doing physical things like swimming, but also running, dancing, cycling – all these things make me feel sexy and confident in my body. I've never been conventionally pretty or particularly slim but I've always felt sexy for me and my partner. I was never prudish and I think that's helped. My mother was always comfortable naked. She probably passed that on.

Sexy is a silly word to me. But to be radiant and gorgeous means to be comfortable on your own skin. To own and love your own at each moment, no matter what that moment is.

Not about those bits. I understand what you mean with that fire. I was lost in love for a couple of years. For me it's playfulness too. Being me. Not more, not less. Being. I feel better in my body than when I was in my twenties. I know who I am, what I need, what I want, what I can give now. It's maybe a sort of self-confidence too?

The inner fire you describe is uber energy and very sexy and self-empowering – and empowering of and for others too. Intensity and stillness: two of the sexiest states I know.

Hadn't really thought of it, but yes! I hated going even in my swimsuit in front of people, but this New Year when everyone was around, I was just like – I'll go first! Look how amazing my body is to be able to do this, come join me!

It's more what ageing does with my mind. It's more unapologetic. I don't see myself through the eyes of others any more. The others stopped messing with my body confidence too: 'Where are your breasts, did you leave them at home?' 'I give a three out of ten.' 'Fat arse.' 'Who wants that?' But I have to say that swimming naked with other naked people is immensely freeing. Everyone has a body, but we are more than our bodies; we are our minds and heart and smile.

We are all bodies, but we are not *just* our bodies; they do not need to define us any more.

TIPS FOR COLD-WATER SWIMMING

These are the things I do, but I know that I am going against advice normally given to people new to outdoor swimming and, in particular, cold-water swimming. However, as you will see, I do take certain precautions every time I plan a dip or swim to mitigate some of the risks I am taking.

- I swim alone, but rarely go out of my depth.
- I dip alone, but mostly in familiar places, and if it doesn't feel right I don't go in.
- I walk to fairly remote places and dip in mountain streams and tarns on my own, often with poor or no mobile signal.

I do all of the above on a regular basis all year round. My logic for doing so is that I want to dip or swim every day and it is not always possible to find a swim buddy, let alone someone to walk and swim with. So, if I did not go on my own, I wouldn't be able to go and it is so important to me to be able to do so.

I *always* err on the side of caution when planning a walking route, or a dip. If it doesn't feel right, or I don't like the walk or water when I get to it, I turn around and walk away. It will be there another day and I want to be there to enjoy it. Or I log it in my head to go back to with a swim buddy.

My go to pieces of kit for cold-water swimming are:

- **Thermos of hot drink:** I warm the flask through first by filling it with boiling water and letting it stand for at least ten minutes. Then I reboil the kettle and make my hot drink, which is usually tea of some sort with no milk, or squash. I need it to be as hot as possible, so adding milk, unless it is hot milk, just would not do the job I need it to do after my dip.
- **Enamel/tin mug:** this is far more effective than the cup on your thermos at warming your hands through as you take sips and enjoy the feeling of steam on your face.
- **Two hats:** one to wear in the water and a dry one to put on afterwards. My favourite kind is merino wool lined with synthetic to stop my head itching! Lightweight, but cosy. I find even if it gets wet in rain or a waterfall, my head stays relatively warm. I often put it straight on after a swim and tuck all my hair up inside so it doesn't drip on me while I get dressed. And then it stays on my head long after I've got home from being out. The bigger, bobble type hats are great, but not as useful as this merino type from Kari Traa, which can be scrunched up in a pocket ready to wear anytime, anywhere.
- **Gloves or mitts:** I use the thermal gloves, which cost about £5 from outdoor shops. They too can get wet and still keep your hands warm and can be worn under mitts. My favourite mitts are from Selkie Swim Company and are thick but lightweight fleece, with two features that make them unique, I believe. They are actually fingerless gloves with a fold-over bit that Velcros back on to the back of your glove when not in use and then pops over your fingers easily. You can get them on cold hands easily, use your fingers to fiddle about with zips and buckles, then pop the fleece over and feel instantly warmer. The other feature is a strip of slightly grippy fabric on the palm of your glove so you can actually drive safely while still wearing them!
- **A mat to stand or sit on:** cold feet, cold bum – neither is pleasant either before or after a dip or swim, especially because the places I go to are often located on the fells or mountains, so there are no convenient flat, clean beaches or benches. Sometimes there are good rocks to perch on, but this is when a lightweight doormat comes in handy for insulating

your bum from the cold, cold rock! I buy £2.99 doormats from Dunelm. They have a rubber backing, but can be put through the washing machine from time to time. I haven't invested in a proper changing mat or anything, maybe I should?!

- **Thermal vest:** particularly for women, I would strongly recommend a sleeveless thermal vest or camisole that you can literally pull on over your feet, pull up your legs and torso so that you are decent and can then put your arms through the armholes or straps. If it's long enough I pull it down and tuck it in my knickers or whatever I'm putting on my bottom half – all body heat sealed in!

The rest of my kit is pretty standard by now with what other cold-water swimmers use. Everyone has their preference of how they get dry, whether that be a microfibre changing robe, like I sometimes use, or a towel. Some people prefer to use their swim cloaks, whichever make they have, to change under, but I find I get in such a tangle and it is quicker for me to rub/pat myself dry, often exposing flesh, and get layers on as quickly as possible. Apres Plunge fleece dungarees (@apresplunge) are my latest favourite piece of all-year-round clothing because they can be pulled on over a wet, cold body and immediately feel cosy and warm. Then I can think about my top half and stand around in just my dungarees (with the bib covering my boobs) untangling my long-sleeved thermal top, or for true minimalist wild swimming I just pull on one of Buffalo Clothing's mountain shirts, which are designed to be worn next to your skin.

If it's really cold or windy, the last piece of clothing I put on is usually my swim cloak to seal in the warming air trapped by the layers of clothing and protect me from any wind or rain.

With practice, you will work out what suits you and your budget. There is so much available on the market now that the choice becomes quite overwhelming. As long as I have my essentials as listed above, I know I will be okay.

Special thanks go to CJB Surf, who were so generous to me when I emailed to ask if they had any C-Skins Legend swim socks available, as mine had worn out and I was going to be needing something to keep my feet unfrozen while I did some proper cold swimming! Not only did a pair of Legend socks arrive, but also C-Skins wired three-millimetre gloves, an amazing Robie Dry-Series swim cloak and a cosy Robie Original-Series change robe. I literally slept in the Dry-Series at the airport in Norway, walked out on to a frozen lake in the dead of night in it and struck up an interesting conversation with airport security at Manchester because of it. Special guests use the Original-Series to walk to and from my Japanese bathtub.

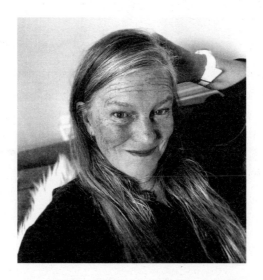

ABOUT THE AUTHOR

Sara Barnes is a self-employed editor based in the English Lake District. She immerses herself in cold water at least once a day, either somewhere in nature, in her outdoor Japanese tub, or further afield to meet other swimmers for a dip in their local waters. She has written for *Outdoor Swimmer* magazine, *The Island Review* and the Outdoor Swimming Society, created and appeared in the environmental film *Spread the Word Not the Weed* and was featured in the 2021 BBC series *The Lakes with Simon Reeve*. As a natural extension of her mini watery narratives on Instagram @bumblebarnes, Sara plans to offer wild water and words retreats, which will combine her qualification as a Level 2 Open Water Swim Coach and her love of writing in nature.